THE Gestational Diabetes Cookbook

THE Gestational Diabetes Cookbook

101 Delicious, Dietitian-Approved Recipes for a Healthy Pregnancy and Baby

SARA RIVERA, RD

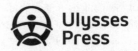

Ulysses Press

Published in the United States by:
ULYSSES PRESS
P.O. Box 3440
Berkeley, CA 94703
www.ulyssespress.com

ISBN: 978-1-61243-868-9
Library of Congress Control Number: 2018959569

Printed in Canada by Marquis Book Printing
10 9 8 7 6 5 4 3 2 1

Acquisitions editor: Bridget Thoreson
Managing editor: Claire Chun
Editor: Renee Rutledge
Proofreader: Shayna Keyles
Front cover design: Rebecca Lown
Interior design: what!design @ whatweb.com
Cover photo: © ESstock/shutterstock.com

Distributed by Publishers Group West

NOTE TO READERS: This book has been written and published strictly for informational and educational purposes only. It is not intended to serve as medical advice or to be any form of medical treatment. You should always consult your physician before altering or changing any aspect of your medical treatment and/or undertaking a diet regimen, including the guidelines as described in this book. Do not stop or change any prescription medications without the guidance and advice of your physician. Any use of the information in this book is made on the reader's good judgment after consulting with his or her physician and is the reader's sole responsibility. This book is not intended to diagnose or treat any medical condition and is not a substitute for a physician.

This book is independently authored and published and no sponsorship or endorsement of this book by, and no affiliation with, any trademarked brands or other products mentioned within is claimed or suggested. All trademarks that appear in ingredient lists and elsewhere in this book belong to their respective owners and are used here for informational purposes only. The author and publisher encourage readers to patronize the quality brands mentioned and pictured in this book.

For Luca, my baby boy. I wrote this book in a very special time of life, the months I carried you. I can't wait to show you the world.

Contents

Chapter Four
Recipes 57

Introduction

There is never a better time to make health a priority than during your pregnancy. Even so, no matter how much effort you put into your health, an unexpected condition can develop at any point in the duration of your pregnancy, whether it's anemia, preeclampsia, infections, or fetal complications. Some conditions are completely out of your control, but some can be managed through diet and lifestyle changes. One such condition is gestational diabetes mellitus (GDM), or gestational diabetes. While it is one of the most dreaded conditions of pregnancy, fortunately, proper nutrition and lifestyle modifications allow you to manage GDM.

GDM, unlike type 1 or type 2 diabetes, can only develop during pregnancy. Gestational diabetes occurs when a pregnant woman's blood sugar levels are elevated because the body produces insufficient insulin, the hormone that reduces blood sugar levels. Uncontrolled blood sugar poses a major risk for mother and baby. Babies of mothers who had uncontrolled blood sugar levels during pregnancy are at a greater risk for developing diabetes and obesity later in life. Babies can also develop an array of complications in the womb if blood sugars are uncontrolled.

These factors are usually what motivate women to control their blood sugars through diet, especially during times of cravings.

Whether you were diagnosed with GDM in your current pregnancy, were diagnosed with it in a previous pregnancy, or are looking to learn about and prevent GDM, you can benefit from reading this book to educate yourself on how to control blood sugar levels and consume a healthy, varied diet. The key to managing GDM is to learn about the healthy foods to consume for you and baby, as well as the foods to limit your intake of.

Carbohydrates are the nutrient that raises blood sugar levels, so it's crucial to follow a carbohydrate-controlled diet plan. You do not want to eliminate carbohydrates from your diet, but should rather focus on incorporating the right kinds of carbohydrates, such as high-fiber and unrefined carbohydrates, as well as consuming as the proper portions. This book will teach you how to do both. You will be able to put your new knowledge to use and discover new foods you will love with the 101 recipes this book contains!

The overall goal when following a carbohydrate-controlled diet is to provide enough nutrients to support your hard-at-work body and meet the needs of your growing baby, all while being mindful to maintain proper blood sugar levels. To do this, your meal plan should consist of small, frequent meals throughout the day. This may sound complicated at first, but after reading the facts and details on GDM and learning how to put together a balanced plate, it will become second nature.

This book will provide background information on what GDM is, including symptoms, causes, and risk factors; complications of gestational diabetes; and a plethora of other useful information. I know you have enough on your plate, whether it's balancing pregnancy and working full time or taking care of toddlers, so the meal planning in this book is simple, and you'll learn how to put together GDM-friendly meals, read Nutrition Facts labels, and create a healthy grocery shopping list with ease.

While GDM is a serious diagnosis and may require medication, sometimes it can be treated naturally with proper nutrition and lifestyle changes alone, if you choose that route. Understanding gestational diabetes and how it affects you and your baby's health can allow you to better grasp the direct impact nutrition has on the condition and equip you to make well-informed decisions.

By following the nutritional guidelines in this cookbook, as well as the delicious and balanced recipes, you will have the necessary tools to stabilize blood sugar levels while ensuring optimal nutrition for your baby. Right now, make this the start of a healthy journey for your growing family.

Chapter One

What Is Gestational Diabetes?

GDM is a common diagnosis for pregnant women. In fact, the Centers for Disease Control and Prevention (CDC) reports the prevalence of GDM among pregnant women is 9.2% and increasing worldwide. Along with the many worries (and joys!) that come with being pregnant, a diagnosis such as GDM can feel crippling. It's important to understand that you likely didn't bring this condition on with your eating habits. In fact, women who are obese or lean can develop gestational diabetes; however, a high body weight is definitely a risk factor for developing GDM. A diagnosis of GDM does not mean you had diabetes prior to pregnancy or that this is a lifelong condition you will have to endure. GDM, diagnosed in pregnancy, can end after giving birth.

GDM is diagnosed when blood sugar, also referred to as blood glucose, is elevated. While the exact cause of GDM is unknown, reduced insulin sensitivity is an identifiable factor. The hormones from the placenta that help the baby develop actually inhibit the mother's insulin from working properly. In other words, the placenta produces hormones that counteract insulin. Insulin, a hormone released by the pancreas, moves glucose into your cells and out of your blood to reduce blood sugar levels. When insulin is not able to perform its job correctly, blood sugar levels remain elevated. This condition is called insulin resistance, or reduced insulin sensitivity, and it tends to begin midpregnancy and worsen as the pregnancy progresses. This is why the glucose tolerance test, a standard test for GDM conducted by all health-care professionals, is not usually given until between weeks 26 and 28 of pregnancy. (The protocol for the test will be discussed shortly.) Insulin resistance generally disappears directly after giving birth.

In normal pregnancies, the body works harder to reduce blood sugar levels, so insulin secretion is increased by 200 to 250%. GDM develops when the body is unable to produce an adequate insulin response to compensate for the hormones counteracting normal insulin resistance. In other words, insulin secretion is increased in normal pregnancies, but not for women with GDM (U. Kampmann et al.).

Symptoms of Gestational Diabetes

The symptoms of GDM are rarely noticed as they're very similar to typical pregnancy symptoms. Fatigue, excessive thirst, and excessive urination are the most common symptoms.

Because symptoms are generally unnoticeable or believed to be normal pregnancy symptoms, women might not realize they have GDM. Women typically don't get diagnosed with gestational diabetes until a routine glucose screening test is conducted.

Glucose Tolerance Test

The routine glucose screening test, also referred to as an oral glucose tolerance test or a sugar test, is usually performed at between 26 and 28 weeks of pregnancy. However, if you have high glucose levels in urine during routine prenatal visits, your doctor or midwife may test you sooner.

One-Hour Glucose Tolerance Test (GTT)

For the one-hour test, you may or may not be asked to fast. A practitioner will have you drink a very sweet beverage called Glucola, which contains 50 grams of glucose, in less than five minutes! Your blood will be drawn one hour later to measure the effect the beverage had on your blood glucose levels. You may or may not get the results right away, and the waiting game is not fun. The desired result is equal to or less than 140 milligrams/deciliter (mg/dL). If your blood glucose levels are higher than this or your practitioner determines you are at risk for GDM, you will be asked to take a three-hour glucose tolerance test.

Three-Hour Glucose Tolerance Test

If you fail the one-hour glucose tolerance test, you will likely need to do the three-hour glucose tolerance test. For the three-hour glucose tolerance test, you will likely be asked to fast for 8 to 14 hours prior to the test. Believe me, I know this is torture for pregnant women, so try to get a morning appointment so you don't feel as if you've gone all day without eating. You may be able to have small amounts of water. Upon coming into the office, you will have your blood drawn prior to drinking Glucola. For the three-hour test, Glucola contains either 75 grams or 100 grams of glucose. Your blood glucose level will be tested one, two, and three hours after drinking Glucola.

Concerns with Glucola

We live in a time of increasing concerns over toxic exposures to new-borns before they even come out of the womb. Some women are highly against drinking Glucola due to the questionable ingredients. Dye-free and BVO-free options are offered, but are still not common today. Some women experience the following symptoms from Glucola: dizziness, headaches, nausea, and vomiting. This makes sense; I mean, it's unlikely you would consume 100 grams of glucose in one sitting.

Many women argue that they would never consume the ingredients in Glucola, especially when pregnant. For women who are focused on eating real, whole, unprocessed foods, and who consciously avoid harmful ingredients, the thought of drinking this "medically approved beverage" could be unsettling. On the other hand, women who do consume excess sugar and processed foods (containing food dyes and dextrose) on a regular basis, such as candy containing the colors of the rainbow, should not necessarily be worried about consuming Glucola once.

Some of the questionable ingredients in Glucola include:

- Brominated vegetable oil, or BVO (an approved flame retardant)

- Modified food starch (a cousin of monosodium glutamate, or MSG)

- Food dyes: FD&C (Food, Drugs & Cosmetics) Yellow#6 and Red#40

- Dextrose (corn sugar; usually derived from GMO corn)

- Sodium hexametaphosphate

- Sodium benzoate

These questionable ingredients are not necessary to include for the effectiveness of the test. What makes the test effective is the sugar content. Glucola contains unnecessary additives that are not well studied in the U.S. and are banned in other countries. So, why is Glucola a standard for most practitioners when there are alternatives? Perhaps this is related to the fact that I am a real food, real ingredients dietitian, but I, for one, did not wish to drink Glucola and was ecstatic when my midwife offered me alternatives before I was even able to ask.

Some alternatives to Glucola are:

- 20 ounces ginger ale

- 16 ounces Coca-Cola

- 14 ounces orange juice

- 10 ounces cranberry juice

- 10 ounces grape juice

- 28 jelly beans

Since jelly beans have been deemed a reliable alternative to Glucola with fewer side effects, a study was conducted on non-pregnant women to test the similarity between the standard 50-gram Glucola beverage and 10 strawberry-flavored Twizzlers. The results indicated that they are an equivalent choice for diabetic screening. They did not study this alternative on pregnant women (D. A. Racusin, et al.).

Another alternative if you refuse to drink Glucola and your practitioner does not allow other beverage alternatives is to test your glucose levels at home four times per day for two weeks. You could pick up supplies for testing over the counter at a pharmacy, or you could request a prescription for a glucometer and test strips from your provider. Depending on your insurance plan, you may or may not have co-pays for the materials. Your provider will likely instruct you to make sure you eat normally during the two weeks to get accurate results, and to test at the following times:

- Test once in the morning upon waking up (this is a fasted test); a normal reading is 60 to 94 mg/dL.

- Test one or two hours after breakfast, lunch, and dinner; a normal reading is 70 to 139 mg/dL.

Call your provider immediately if you get an elevated reading.

You may be reading this book after already having taken the test. However, should you have more children, you will be able to use this information to make an informed decision about which method you choose for your next glucose tolerance test. When the test is brought up in conversation, or you are asked by newly pregnant mothers, you will be able to offer advice and information they are unaware of.

Overall, consuming this drink one time will not likely cause long-term health issues, but hopefully the medical community and conventional practitioners will continue to research and develop a cleaner drink or allow all women to use food and beverage alternatives for the test—especially the healthier options such as orange or cranberry juice.

Causes and Risk Factors of GDM

There's no definitive answer as to why some pregnant women develop gestational diabetes and others do not. As aforementioned, the hormones produced by the placenta inhibit insulin from properly performing its job to lower blood sugar levels. As the placenta continues to grow as pregnancy progresses, the number of insulin-counteracting hormones rises. This is another reason why gestational diabetes usually develops and is diagnosed beginning around the twenty-sixth week of pregnancy.

The following indicators, along with a maternal age of over 25 years, are common risk factors for pregnant women to develop gestational diabetes:

Body mass index (BMI). BMI is a measure of weight relative to height. Gestational diabetes is diagnosed in both women with BMIs in the normal and obese categories, but the pathophysiology differs between the two groups:

- **BMI in obese category (BMI = 30 or higher).** Obesity prior to pregnancy and at 28 weeks pregnant is correlated to increased insulin resistance. Adipose tissue (stored fat tissue) is believed to cause insulin resistance. If you were overweight pre-pregnancy, you likely had insulin resistance, but may not have known if you didn't get routine blood work conducted. During pregnancy, the insulin resistance is amplified.

- **BMI in normal category (BMI = 18.5 to 24.9).** Women in this category can develop insulin resistance during pregnancy, despite a normal BMI. However, lean women typically do not have the pre-pregnancy insulin resistance found in obese women.

Ethnicity. The prevalence of GDM is higher in women who are African American, Hispanic American, Native American, Pacific Islander, and South or East Asian, compared to non-Hispanic white women.

History of diabetes. A family history of diabetes increases GDM risk, such as having a family member with type 1 or type 2 diabetes. Also, gestational diabetes in prior pregnancies or prediabetes prior to pregnancy increases risk for GDM. Prediabetes is a condition characterized by slightly elevated blood glucose levels, which indicates risk for progression to type 2 diabetes. Prediabetes is diagnosed when hemoglobin A1C level is between 5.7 to 6.4%. The hemoglobin A1C test reflects your blood sugar average from the past three months by measuring the percentage of hemoglobin that is coated with sugar. Hemoglobin is a protein found in red blood cells that carries oxygen throughout the body and gives blood its red color.

Polycystic ovary syndrome (PCOS). Fifty percent of women with PCOS have coexisting metabolic syndrome, which includes insulin resistance.

Women with PCOS are at greater risk for developing type 2 diabetes. This is why they are typically considered high risk during pregnancy and therefore are instructed to follow a strict diet and are advised not to gain excess weight (M.-L. Pan et al.).

Complications

During pregnancy, stillbirths were previously found to be a risk and complication for women with gestational diabetes. However, presently the risk of stillbirths is lower than previous times, likely due to increased monitoring and treatment of GDM. On the following pages, I'll discuss potential complications during pregnancy, delivery, and postpartum.

Hypertensive Disorders

Hypertensive disorders can occur during pregnancy. Women with GDM are at higher risk for developing them. Hypertensive disorders range from mild to severe in the order of gestational hypertension, preeclampsia, and eclampsia.

Gestational hypertension. Gestational hypertension occurs when a woman who had normal blood pressure pre-pregnancy develops high blood pressure when she is more than 20 weeks pregnant. Blood pressure usually normalizes 12 weeks postpartum. Gestational hypertension can be difficult to recognize as there are usually no symptoms associated with it, similar to GDM. Usually, the mother and baby are unharmed from the mild high blood pressure. However, gestational hypertension progresses to preeclampsia in 15 to 25% of women, and this is when complications can occur (P. Saudan, et al.).

Preeclampsia. Also referred to as toxemia, this can occur during the second half of pregnancy and includes high blood pressure at or greater than 140/90 millimeters of mercury (mmHg), increased swelling, excess protein in the urine, and an abnormal development of the placenta. Preeclampsia can cause serious or life-threatening conditions for both you and baby. There is no cure for preeclampsia, except to give birth, which is why some doctors advise their patients to give birth at 37 weeks of pregnancy. However, some women go into unplanned preterm labor, which is birth before 37 weeks.

Eclampsia. This occurs when the blood pressure is so severe than it can affect the pregnant mother's brain function. This can cause seizures or the onset of a coma. Women with either preeclampsia or eclampsia can suffer damage to the liver and blood cells. This condition is known as HELLP syndrome. HELLP stands for:

H   Hemolysis: oxygen-carrying red blood cells break down

EL   Elevated Liver enzymes: liver damage

LP   Low Platelet count: the cells that stop bleeding, platelets, have a low count

Complications during Delivery

Gestational diabetes may increase your chance of having a cesarean section (C-section) due to fetal macrosomia. Fetal macrosomia is a term used to describe newborns with birth weights larger than average, at greater than 8 pounds and 13 ounces (regardless of gestational age). The increased body fat is directly related to the excess sugar in mom's body. Baby absorbs excess sugar that your body cannot metabolize. You can read more about this on page 29. A study found a direct correlation between C-section rates and women with gestational diabetes: 19.5% of women with gestational diabetes had a non-elective C-section rate compared to 13.5% for non-diabetic women (U. Kampmann, et al.).

Shoulder dystocia is another complication that can occur during delivery. Shoulder dystocia is a term used to describe obstructed labor where the shoulders fail to deliver after the head. There is an association between increased fetal size and the risk of shoulder dystocia.

Postpartum Type 2 Diabetes

Gestational diabetes can predispose you to other disorders postpartum. For example, you are more at risk for developing type 2 diabetes later in life. Your blood sugars may normalize shortly after delivery, but this does not exclude you from an increased risk for type 2 diabetes development. It's crucial to monitor blood sugar levels postpartum by getting routine blood work conducted and getting a yearly fasting glucose test done.

Type 2 diabetes is the most common type of diabetes. The other types of diabetes include type 1 and GDM. Type 1 diabetes differs from type 2 diabetes because in patients with type 1 diabetes, the body does not produce insulin. Type 1 diabetes is classified as an autoimmune condition in which one's body attacks the insulin-producing cells of the pancreas, which are called beta cells. When you consume carbohydrates, your body breaks them down in the form of glucose. Without insulin, sugar remains elevated in the blood. Patients with type 1 diabetes require taking insulin daily in the form of an injection or an insulin pump. An insulin pump delivers insulin through a catheter that is placed under the skin and mimics the work of a pancreas by delivering small amounts of insulin throughout the day, much like a true pancreas does.

In type 2 diabetes, your body is able to produce insulin, but either not enough is made or the insulin is not used efficiently, which is referred to as insulin resistance. When the body's cells are constantly being fed sugar, which is common in the Standard American Diet (SAD), they become desensitized to insulin's blood sugar–lowering effects. Think about it like this: the cells that "open the door" and take the sugar out of the blood are constantly bombarded with insulin so they no longer do what they are supposed to, which is why blood sugar levels remain high. Type 2 diabetes is both preventable and reversible; diet and lifestyle are two important factors. Eating balanced meals consisting of unprocessed carbohydrates, protein, and healthy fats, and limiting added sugar intake can decrease your risk of developing type 2 diabetes. With uncontrolled blood sugars, patients with type 2 diabetes are required to take medication. With very uncontrolled blood sugars, insulin therapy may be introduced.

Having uncontrolled blood sugars for an extended time can lead to a plethora of complications, including diabetic retinopathy (a complication of diabetes that affects the eyes), heart disease, kidney disease, and nerve damage that can lead to neuropathy (weakness, numbness, and pain, usually in the hands and feet).

Postpartum Cardiovascular Disease

The risk of cardiovascular disease (CVD), otherwise known as heart disease, is approximately 70% higher in women with previously diagnosed GDM compared to women without GDM history. Many conditions fall under the umbrella of CVD, including heart attacks, strokes, heart failure, arrhythmia (abnormal heartbeat), and aortic stenosis (narrowing of the large blood vessel that branches off of the heart). The onset of CVD is attributed to the development of type 2 diabetes, increased risk of metabolic syndrome, and/or vascular dysfunction. Vascular dysfunction includes dysfunction of large arteries (due to hardening of the arteries, also referred to as atherosclerosis), microcirculation, and endothelial dysfunction. Thus, preventing type 2 diabetes can reduce the risk of CVD development.

Another way to reduce the risk of CVD development is to make healthy lifestyle changes: Quit smoking, moderate alcohol consumption, eat a balanced diet, increase fruit and vegetable intake, limit processed foods, reduce excessive dining out, prioritize physical activity, achieve a healthy weight, reduce stress levels, and, overall, take care of yourself mentally and physically. In a nutshell, living a healthy lifestyle after pregnancy can prevent the onset, or delay the progression of, nutrition-related diseases.

Postpartum Metabolic Syndrome

Metabolic syndrome is a cluster of metabolic disorders that puts one at a high risk for developing cardiovascular disease and type 2 diabetes.

Metabolic syndrome is diagnosed if you have three or more of the following metabolic disorders:

- Central or abdominal obesity (this is measured by waist circumference)

  » Men: waist greater than 40 inches

  » Women: waist greater than 35 inches

- Triglycerides greater than or equal to 150 milligrams per deciliter of blood (mg/dL)

- HDL cholesterol

  » Men: less than 40 mg/dL

  » Women: less than 50 mg/dL

- Blood pressure greater than or equal to 130/85 mmHg

- Fasting glucose greater than or equal to 100 mg/dL

The prevalence of metabolic syndrome tends to be higher in women who previously had GDM. For example, a study demonstrated that the prevalence of metabolic syndrome three months postpartum was 10% in women without blood sugar issues, 17.6% in women with impaired glucose tolerance during pregnancy, and 20% in women with a history of GDM (U. Kampmann, et al.). Monitoring your risk for metabolic syndrome, and beginning interventions through lifestyle modifications and diet, is key to preventing diabetes and cardiovascular disease.

How GDM Affects Baby

You now know how GDM can affect your health, but learning how it can affect your baby's health may be your true motivator in making healthy lifestyle changes. Fortunately, GDM does not cause birth defects due to the fact that GDM is diagnosed later in pregnancy, after the baby has already been developed. During the time when baby's organs are developing, the mother usually has normal blood glucose levels. However, poorly controlled GDM can affect your baby in other ways. In short, with GDM, the high blood glucose crosses through the placenta to the baby, which raises the baby's blood glucose levels. The baby's pancreas then works hard to make extra insulin to lower the blood glucose. While insulin is a hormone that lowers blood glucose, it also stores unneeded carbohydrates as fat. Remember, insulin is a fat-storing hormone. With GDM, since the baby is getting more energy than it needs from carbohydrates, the extra energy is stored as fat, which could lead to macrosomia (a large baby). As you have learned, this could lead to a C-section being the only delivery option.

Babies of mothers with GDM are more at risk of developing metabolic diseases later in life, such as obesity, type 2 diabetes, and metabolic syndrome. Although this concept has not been thoroughly studied, emerging research shows that high insulin levels in fetuses could possibly modify growth and future metabolism of the fetus. Furthermore, if you were to look at a graph of birth weight and the increased risk of type 2 diabetes, it would be U-shaped. This means that infants with both decreased and increased birth weights are at higher risk of developing type 2 diabetes, whereas infants with a normal birth weight are not at risk.

Another effect of GDM on newborns is the possibility of very low blood glucose levels at birth, which is also referred to as hypoglycemia. (Remember, hypoglycemia means low blood glucose and hyperglycemia means high blood glucose.) Hypoglycemia occurs in newborns when the mother's blood glucose levels have been consistently high. This is because the fetus has high levels of insulin as the body works to reduce blood glucose levels. After birth, the baby continues to have high insulin levels, although there are no longer high levels of glucose coming from his or her mother; thus, the newborn's blood glucose becomes very low. If a baby is born hypoglycemic, glucose may be given through an IV to raise blood glucose levels.

Not only can insulin cause the baby to become overweight and hypo-glycemic, but it can also lead to breathing problems. Too much insulin in the baby's body can delay surfactant production, which is necessary for lungs to mature so baby can breathe on his or her own outside the womb.

Conventional Treatments for GDM

Several medications are prescribed to women with GDM. When lifestyle interventions are inadequate and blood sugar is not well controlled, insulin therapy may be introduced, such as injected insulin or an insulin pump. Be sure to always advocate for yourself, as some practitioners will encourage you to take insulin without trying lifestyle modifications first. Insulin is not dangerous to take as it does not cross the placenta and, therefore, does not harm baby. However, although it is considered safe, it can be difficult, and quite frankly annoying, for the mother to administer. If your provider recommends insulin, you will need to be educated on how to safely administer it. While pricking your finger throughout the day isn't quite enjoyable, sometimes it is necessary to help normalize blood sugar when lifestyle modifications are not sufficient.

Another conventional treatment is oral medication. Oral medication has not been approved for GDM in all countries; however, in the U.S., gly-buride and metformin are commonly prescribed. Both medications are oral antidiabetic agents that can be used as an alternative to insulin. Some studies show that metformin crosses the placenta, which could potentially affect baby's metabolism, but further studies need to be conducted. The safety of these drugs is still being researched, so be sure to speak with your provider about the benefits and risks of medications.

Natural Treatments for GDM

Lifestyle change is a cornerstone in the natural treatment of GDM and is typically the primary intervention before medication is necessary to introduce. Lifestyle changes include a combination of nutrition counseling and education by a registered dietitian or certified diabetes educator, physical activity, and self-monitoring of blood glucose. The nutrition protocol for GDM will be reviewed shortly.

Self-monitoring of blood glucose includes testing blood sugar frequently throughout the day, before and after meals, by drawing blood from your finger and placing it on a strip that displays the blood glucose number. Keeping a blood sugar and diet log is crucial to help you identify foods that cause a spike in your blood sugar and certain times of day when your blood sugar tends to be elevated (such as the morning). With this data, you will be better able to administer the appropriate amount of insulin, if you are taking insulin, or you will understand which foods best help to keep your blood sugar within the appropriate range.

Vitamin D

Growing evidence suggests a possible association between vitamin D deficiency and GDM, maternal obesity, and adverse maternal, neonatal, and infant outcomes.

The science behind the association of vitamin D and GDM, in regard to molecular and cellular mechanisms, is only partly understood. Further evidence needs to be obtained to determine whether or not vitamin D supplementation can reduce risk of developing GDM or improve blood sugar control in women with GDM. Regardless, optimal vitamin D levels are crucial. It's likely that your prenatal supplement does not contain an adequate amount of vitamin D. The American Pregnancy Association reports that intaking 4,000 international units (IU) of vitamin D per day has the greatest benefits in preventing preterm labor and birth as well as infections. Most prenatal supplements have about 400 IU of vitamin D, so I encourage you to take an additional vitamin D supplement.

Vitamin D is beneficial for both you and baby. For you, it supports immune function, healthy cell division, and bone health. It also aids in the absorption of calcium and phosphorous. For baby, vitamin D supports healthy bone development.

In my private practice, about 80% of my patients are vitamin D deficient, especially in the colder months. Vitamin D deficiency is very common among Americans. If your doctor or midwife tells you that you are deficient in vitamin D, take it seriously and take your supplements as directed.

Calcium

Calcium is another nutrient of concern in regard to GDM. According to research, higher dietary calcium intake (from food, not supplements) is shown to reduce the risk of GDM development. In a study published in *Public Health Nutrition*, women who consumed higher amounts of dietary calcium had 42% lower risk of GDM. For women with a calcium intake below 1,200 milligrams per day, a 200 milligram increase per day was associated with a 22% reduction in GDM risk. This suggests that higher levels of calcium intake are associated with lower GDM risk.

Calcium is crucial during pregnancy because adequate intake reduces your risk of developing hypertension and preeclampsia. Calcium is a nutrient that supports several systems in the body, including the musculoskeletal, nervous, and circulatory systems. Your baby needs calcium to build strong bones, teeth, nerves, and muscles. It also helps baby grow a healthy heart. If you are not intaking enough calcium during pregnancy, baby can actually draw it out from your bones, which increases your risk for developing osteoporosis later in life. Eat calcium-rich foods such as yogurt or kefir, cheese, sardines, cooked kale, broccoli, bok choy, okra, and almonds. Ask your doctor if calcium supplements are necessary.

Stress Management

Many of us are stressed, yet we do not take into account how much it directly impacts our health and well-being. Stress can directly affect your hormone levels and, furthermore, disrupt your blood sugar levels. Find the right tools to manage your stress levels, such as yoga, meditation, walking, journaling, self-care, or alone time. Giving yourself as little as 20 minutes per day can help reduce stress levels, which is not only important for you, but for baby as well. A life-changing event, pregnancy can be a high-stress time for some pregnant women. Stress is not to be ignored; it is crucial to take the necessary steps to manage it.

Women with GDM, in particular those who are on insulin, may have stress related to dietary management. In other words, they can become confused about what to eat or are fearful that their diet will cause complications with their baby. To ease stress related to GDM, be sure to seek counseling from a registered dietitian to ensure you're consuming the right balance of foods. Having an extra set of eyes on your food intake, or the extra support alone, can help you find comfort with your diet and reduce stress levels.

Chapter Two

Nutrition Protocol for GDM

Foods are made up of carbohydrates, fats, and protein. These nutrients are also referred to as macronutrients. Carbohydrates make up a huge chunk of our food supply, including:

- Fruit

- Starchy veggies: corn, peas, potatoes, plantains, yucca, pumpkin, legumes (black, red, kidney beans, lentils, edamame)

- Non-starchy veggies: all other vegetables, such as broccoli, peppers, onions, and mushrooms

- Grains and breads (starches): bread, rice, pasta, crackers, couscous, hot and cold cereal

- Milk and sweetened yogurts

- Sweets and desserts

Carbohydrates are the only macronutrient to raise blood glucose levels, as they turn into sugar in the body when digested. Carbohydrates are an important part of a healthy diet, particularly fruits and vegetables, so they *must not be eliminated from your diet.* Healthy carbohydrates provide vitamins, minerals, and fiber. The portion of carbohydrates you consume at meals and snacks is the most important factor in controlling blood glucose levels. Carb counting is an excellent tool to help you successfully consume an appropriate amount of carbohydrates. The protocol for carb counting begins on page 47.

Nutrition Facts Label

In 2016, the FDA announced that there would be an updated Nutrition Facts label for packaged foods due to updated scientific information, such as the association between diet and chronic nutrition-related diseases; obesity and heart disease is one example. The FDA developed the new label to help consumers make better-informed food choices. The original compliance date for food manufacturers was July 26, 2018. However, the FDA has extended the compliance date to January 1, 2020 for manufacturers with $10 million or more in annual food sales and January 1, 2021 for manufacturers with less than $10 million in food sales. Some manufacturers have already begun utilizing the new Nutrition Facts label, such as KIND.

The new label contains:

- A larger font size for calories, servings per container, and the serving size

- Bolded number of calories and serving size

- The amount of vitamin D, calcium, iron, and potassium (nutrients Americans are commonly deficient in)

- Added sugars in grams and as percent daily value (%DV)

When reading a food label, first look at the serving size. All of the information on the label is based on this portion. What's most important for you, having GDM, is to review the total grams of carbohydrates in the serving size. If you are consuming a food product that is already using the new Nutrition Facts label, review the section that says "added sugars" under "total sugars." You want to limit "added sugars" as much as possible.

Old label

Nutrition Facts	
Serving Size 2/3 cup (55g)	
Servings Per Container About 8	
Amount Per Serving	
Calories 230	Calories from Fat 72
	% Daily Value*
Total Fat 8g	12%
Saturated Fat 1g	5%
Trans Fat 0g	
Cholesterol 0mg	0%
Sodium 160mg	7%
Total Carbohydrate 37g	12%
Dietary Fiber 4g	16%
Sugars 12g	
Protein 3g	
Vitamin A	10%
Vitamin C	8%
Calcium	20%
Iron	45%

* Percent Daily Values are based on a 2,000 calorie diet. Your daily value may be higher or lower depending on your calorie needs.

	Calories:	2,000	2,500
Total Fat	Less than	65g	80g
Sat Fat	Less than	20g	25g
Cholesterol	Less than	300mg	300mg
Sodium	Less than	2,400mg	2,400mg
Total Carbohydrate		300g	375g
Dietary Fiber		25g	30g

New label

Nutrition Facts	
8 servings per container	
Serving size	**2/3 cup (55g)**
Amount per serving	
Calories	**230**
	% Daily Value*
Total Fat 8g	10%
Saturated Fat 1g	5%
Trans Fat 0g	
Cholesterol 0mg	0%
Sodium 160mg	7%
Total Carbohydrate 37g	13%
Dietary Fiber 4g	14%
Total Sugars 12g	
Includes 10g Added Sugars	20%
Protein 3g	
Vitamin D 2mcg	10%
Calcium 260mg	20%
Iron 8mg	45%
Potassium 235mg	6%

* The % Daily Value (DV) tells you how much a nutrient in a serving of food contributes to a daily diet. 2,000 calories a day is used for general nutrition advice.

Added Sugars

The old Nutrition Facts label does not break down the "sugars" category, so it's unknown whether you are consuming naturally occurring sugar (from fruit, for example) or added sugar. The best thing you can do is review the ingredients list and find the source of sugar. A general guideline is to avoid all added sugars and choose foods with at least 4 grams of fiber. Fiber is important because it slows down the emptying of your stomach and, thus, slows the absorption of carbohydrates. This is because fiber absorbs water and forms a gel in your gestational tract (GI tract). When choosing starches to put on your plate, choose high-fiber carbohydrates to prevent blood sugar spikes. A list of good high-fiber carbohydrate options will be reviewed shortly.

Sugar goes by many names in an ingredients list. Get into the habit of not only reviewing the grams of carbohydrates, but also reviewing the ingredients list. If the ingredients list contains some variation of the word "sugar," "juice," or "syrup," such as "cane juice" or "beet sugar," then it is just another word for sugar. The list below will show you other common words used in the ingredients list for added sugar. Food companies are quite tricky—over time you will learn they may have four to five different words for sugar spread throughout the ingredients list.

Names for added sugar include:

- Agave

- Caramel

- Crystalline fructose

- Fructose

- Honey

- Molasses

- Sorghum

- Sucrose

- Treacle

Sugar alcohols (which you can identify because they end in "OL") are harder for the body to digest and are not completely absorbed, so they do not raise blood sugar as much as regular carbohydrates do. In fact, sugar alcohols can cause digestive issues in some people, including bloating, gas, cramping, and diarrhea. Some providers suggest subtracting half of the grams of sugar alcohol from the total grams of carbohydrates but others suggest not counting sugar alcohols toward total grams of carbohydrates. Clarify with your dietitian or certified diabetes educator (CDE) how you should count sugar alcohols. Sugar alcohols include:

- Erythritol

- Maltitol

- Mannitol

- Sorbitol

- Xylitol

Artificial sweeteners include:

- Aspartame (NutraSweet, Equal)

- Neotame (NutraSweet)

- Saccharin (Sweet'n Low)

- Sucralose (Splenda)

Safe natural sweeteners (which do not impact blood sugar) include:

- Stevia

- Swerve

- Lakanto maple syrup

- Truvia

There is no one-size-fits-all approach for the amount of carbohydrates to consume per serving. After you are diagnosed with GDM, your provider will refer you to a registered dietitian or certified diabetes educator to develop an individualized meal plan for you. It would be best if your dietitian can make you a menu based on your individual food preferences, so that it is a more realistic plan for you.

Also, based on how carbohydrates affect your individual blood glucose, your dietitian or certified diabetes educator will decide how many carbohydrate servings you should consume at meals and at snacks to keep your blood glucose within the target range. For example, one woman with GDM may have a larger spike in blood glucose after eating a piece of bread than another woman with GDM. There are certain factors that play a role in how foods affect your individual blood sugar, including medications, physical activity, and metabolic responses. It's important to check your blood sugar levels and keep a log of both your blood sugar and food so that your dietitian can develop a plan that best suits your needs. Keeping a log will also help your dietitian determine where changes in the plan may be needed at follow-up visits.

The Plate Method

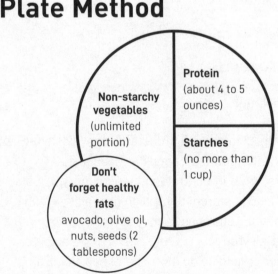

Non-starchy vegetables (unlimited portion)

Protein (about 4 to 5 ounces)

Starches (no more than 1 cup)

Don't forget healthy fats avocado, olive oil, nuts, seeds (2 tablespoons)

The image above gives you an idea of how your plate should look to ensure you are consuming a balanced meal and hitting all the food groups. The goal is to fill half your plate with non-starchy vegetables (unlimited portion), a quarter of the plate with protein (about 4 to 5 ounces), and a quarter of the plate with starches (about a fist size, or no more than 1 cup). Remember, starches are very important to portion control. The second image of the healthy fats is there to remind you that it's crucial to include healthy fats in your diet. A good rule of thumb is to add at least 2 tablespoons of healthy fats to each meal. Healthy fats aid in slowing down the absorption of carbohydrates and will keep you satiated longer. Not to mention, they are excellent to consume as they support baby's brain and eye development.

You can have meals that do not have a starch source, especially if you aren't very hungry. The two most important foods to have on your plate are a source of protein and a non-starchy vegetable. Non-starchy vegetables, although a carbohydrate, have very limited impact on blood sugar levels and, thus, do not need to be restricted to 1 cup. In fact, treat them as if they were not a carbohydrate, and make them the biggest portion on your plate.

As you can see, a diet can contain many different carbohydrates, and all will impact your blood sugar differently. For example, a large spinach salad with tomatoes, onions, and cucumbers topped with grilled shrimp will have very little impact on your blood sugar levels compared to white pasta and marinara sauce. The pasta dish will greatly impact your blood sugar levels due to the refined carbohydrate (white pasta) and lack of protein or healthy fats.

Many of us are used to making the starch the biggest portion on the plate, whether it's rice, potatoes, or pasta. Making changes to your starch portion is the first step in controlling blood sugars. It's also crucial to choose the *right kind* of starch (think: high fiber and unrefined). There are two lists below of good starches to choose from: Starchy Vegetables and High-Fiber Starches. On your plate, starchy vegetables and high-fiber starches, together, should be no more than 1 cup. For example, if you are eating potatoes and peas, the portion is 1 cup total rather than 1 cup each.

Many people are reluctant to make the switch from white pasta to a healthier, high-fiber pasta. However, just because you didn't enjoy whole wheat pasta doesn't mean you won't enjoy brown rice pasta or chickpea pasta. It also takes your taste buds some time to adjust to new food, so I encourage you to continue trying a food even if you didn't like it the first time. Perhaps you tried chickpea pasta once and didn't enjoy it. Try it again with a different sauce or different flavors. The only way to expand your palate and eat a variety of foods is to continue trying new ones.

And, I know, I get it, sometimes in pregnancy, you want what you want. *You're craving a bowl of white pasta with marinara sauce.* If you cannot shake the craving, make sure to have an appropriate portion and include healthy fat or protein to prevent blood sugar spikes.

In order for you to be able to build a healthy, balanced, GDM-friendly plate, here's a breakdown of the various food groups along with the recommended serving size per plate.

Protein

Serving size: 4 to 5 ounces; does not impact blood sugar levels

For a complete list, refer to the back of the book on page 171.

- Beef
- Bison
- Burgers: beef, veggie, chicken, turkey
- Chicken
- Cottage cheese
- Eggs
- Fish
- Ground meat: chicken, turkey, beef
- Lamb
- Sausages
- Seafood
- Turkey
- Plain Greek yogurt
- Pork

- Sliced deli meat (be sure to heat it to avoid potential listeria contamination)
- Venison
- Whey

Fat

Serving size: at least 2 tablespoons; does not impact blood sugar levels

- Avocado
- Butter
- Cheese
- Coconut milk
- Cream
- Ghee
- Mayonnaise
- Nuts
- Nut butters: peanut, almond, cashew
- Oils: olive, avocado, coconut
- Olives
- Seeds

Non-Starchy Vegetables

Serving size: unlimited portion; has minimal impact on blood sugar levels

- Alfalfa sprouts
- Artichokes
- Arugula
- Asparagus
- Beans: green, Italian, wax
- Bean sprouts
- Beets
- Broccoli
- Broccoli rabe
- Brussels sprouts
- Cabbage: bok choy, Chinese, green
- Carrots
- Cauliflower
- Celery
- Collard greens
- Cucumbers

- Eggplant
- Green onions (or scallions)
- Kale
- Leeks
- Lettuce and salad greens
- Mung beans
- Mushrooms
- Mustard greens
- Okra
- Onions

- Peppers
- Radishes
- Sauerkraut
- Sea vegetables
- Spinach
- Swiss chard
- Turnips
- Turnip greens
- Water chestnuts
- Zucchini

Starchy Vegetables

Serving size: no more than 1 cup; impacts blood sugar levels

- Legumes (black beans, kidney beans, chickpeas, lentils, red beans)
- Parsnips
- Peas
- Plantains

- Potatoes
- Pumpkin
- Squash
- Yams
- Yucca

High-Fiber Starches

Serving size: no more than 1 cup cooked; impacts blood sugar levels

- Amaranth
- Barley
- Bulgur

- Corn
- Ezekiel bread
- Farro

- Millet
- Muesli
- Oats
- Pastas: black bean, red lentil, brown rice, chickpea, Einkorn

- Quinoa
- Rice (brown, wild)
- Spelt
- Teff
- Tortillas (sprouted grain)

Starches to Avoid
Avoid these foods: greatly impacts blood sugar levels

- White pasta (½ cup)
- White bread (1 slice), bagels (½), wraps (1 wrap)

- White rice (½ cup)
- Cereals (⅔ cup)

Fruits
Spread your fruit intake out throughout the day to help stabilize blood sugar levels. Fruits are an excellent snack choice, especially when paired with a healthy fat or protein to help slow the absorption of the sugar. Review the fruits below and be sure to always pair a healthy fat or protein with the higher-carb fruits. Avoid fruit juices, as they do not contain fiber and have a high sugar content.

Lower-Carb Fruits
Serving size: 1 small piece or 1 cup; little to moderate impact on blood sugar levels

- Berries (raspberries, blackberries, strawberries, blueberries, cranberries)
- Cantaloupe
- Cherries
- Clementines

- Figs
- Grapefruits
- Guavas
- Kiwis
- Lemons

- Limes
- Nectarines
- Papayas
- Peaches

- Plums
- Rhubarbs
- Tangerines
- Tomatoes

Higher-Carb Fruits
Serving size: ½ cup; may cause a spike in blood sugar level

- Apples
- Apricots
- Bananas
- Dried fruits
- Grapes
- Mangos

- Oranges
- Pears
- Pineapples
- Pomegranates
- Watermelons

Adequate water intake is also very important with both pregnancy and GDM. Drink at least *eight glasses of water daily*. Drinking plenty of water is important in building body fluids, proper digestion, and blood circulation. Extra water also aids the kidneys in expelling extra sugar from the blood.

Be Realistic

Aside from following the portions in the plate method, it's important to make sure you are realistic about your meal planning. You need to choose foods that you will be satisfied with and enjoy. If you were diagnosed around week 28 of pregnancy, you could potentially be eating a carbohydrate-controlled plan for 14 more weeks. The more content you are with your meals, the more likely you are to comply with the diet. The good news is, you may find yourself enjoying some of the new foods and notice a positive difference in your energy levels. Although the GDM diet is short-term, know that some of the changes you make and what you learn along the way can be sustainable and helpful for your future health. For example, if non-starchy veggies were not a priority on your plate before following the GDM diet, afterward, you may get so used to making veggies a part of your meals that you will continue to do so.

Carb Counting

Some dietitians will instruct you to count grams of carbs at each meal and snack, while some may suggest carb counting. Carbohydrates are measured in grams (g). Essentially, counting grams of carbs and carb counting are the same thing because 15 grams of carbs = 1 carb count. Other dietitians may simply have you follow portion guidelines, such as consuming no more than 1 cup of carbohydrates per meal. The method that makes the most sense to you, and is easiest for you to follow, is the best option.

Below is an example of the three different options:

Different Ways of Counting Carbs

Meal	Carbs/meal	Carb count/meal	Portions/meal
Breakfast 8:00 a.m.	15–30 grams	1–2	½ cup carbs
Snack 10:00 a.m.	15–20 grams	1	1 cup low-carb fruit or ½ cup non-starchy vegetables
Lunch 12:30 p.m.	30–45 grams	2–3	1 cup carbs
Snack 2:30 p.m.	15–20 grams	1	1 cup low-carb fruit or ½ cup non-starchy vegetables
Dinner 5:00 p.m.	30–45 grams	2–3	1 cup carbs
Snack 7:00 p.m.	15 grams or less	1	1 cup low-carb fruit or ½ cup non-starchy vegetables

Regardless of the method, measuring your food and understanding proper portions will help you control your blood sugar. You may have several carbohydrate servings in one sitting, based on your meal plan. For example, your meal plan may allow for 30 or 45 grams of carbs at lunch and dinner. Remember, you can identify how many grams of carbohydrates are in foods by checking the Nutrition Facts label on packaged foods. If one serving of chips contains 30 grams of carbohydrates, that would be 2 carb servings. For foods without the Nutrition Facts labels, such as fruits and vegetables, measuring your food with portions is the best way to understand how many carbohydrates to consume.

Below is a general guideline for grams of carbohydrates in fruits and vegetables. You will find that the serving sizes are smaller than the plate method mentioned previously. However, you are able to have multiple servings depending on how your blood sugar is impacted. For example, you may find your blood sugar is stable after 2 portions of starchy vegetables (for a total of 1 cup) and thus there is no reason to limit your intake to ½ cup. The chart provides the carbohydrate grams per serving. The amount of servings you can have is individualized and based on how you metabolize the food (and ultimately your blood sugar readings).

Carbohydrates per Gram in Fruits and Vegetables

Food	Serving Size	Carbohydrate grams per serving
Starchy Vegetables	3-ounce baked potato ½ cup mashed potatoes ½ cup beans ½ cup peas	15
Non-Starchy Vegetables	1 cup cooked (broccoli, asparagus, etc.) 2 cups raw vegetables (romaine lettuce, spinach)	10 to 15
Fruits and Fruit Juices	1 small fresh fruit ½ cup unsweetened fruit juice (4 ounces) 2 tablespoons dried fruit	15

Range of Carbohydrates per Carb Count

Total Carb Grams	Carb Count
0 to 5	0
6 to 10	½
11 to 20	1
21 to 25	1½
26 to 35	2
36 to 40	2½
41 to 50	3
51 to 55	3½
56 to 65	4

Fiber Is Your Friend

The more fiber a food contains, the less your blood sugar will spike. For example, if a food contains more than 5 grams of dietary fiber, you can subtract one half of the fiber grams from the total carbohydrate grams.

Example: Split Peas

Carbohydrates: 19g
Fiber: 7g

Subtract half of the total fiber because it is over 5 grams. Subtracting 3½ grams of fiber (half of 7 grams of fiber) from 19 grams of carbs = 15½ grams of carbs. Look at the chart above and you will see 15½ grams of carbs falls into the category of 1 carb count.

Sample Meal Plan

Overnight, hormones tend to make blood sugars higher in the morning, so a smaller amount of carbohydrates should be consumed in the evening. Avoid fruit for breakfast, as it is not metabolized well in the morning. Bedtime snacks can help you avoid nighttime hypoglycemia, especially if you are on long-acting insulin.

Sample Meal Plan

Breakfast 8:00 a.m. (1–2 carb counts = 15–30 carb grams)	2 whole eggs scrambled with tomatoes, peppers, and onions 1 slice Ezekiel flax toast, buttered 1 cup coffee with regular cream and Stevia
Snack 10:00 a.m. (1 carb count = 15 carb grams)	1 cup cucumber/sliced green peppers 2 tablespoons hummus
Lunch 12:30 p.m. (2–3 carb counts = 30–45 carb grams)	1 turkey burger, bunless ½ cup quinoa 1 cup sautéed mushrooms and onions 1 cup berries
Snack 2:30 p.m. (1 carb count = 15 carb grams)	1 apple 2 tablespoons no-added sugar peanut butter
Dinner 5:00 p.m. (2–3 carb counts = 30–45 carb grams)	4 ounces salmon ½ sweet potato with 1 tablespoon butter 1 cup broccoli
Snack 7:00 p.m. (1 carb count = 15 carb grams)	1 cup plain Greek yogurt with 1 tablespoon chia seeds or ground flax seeds

Meal Timing

As you can see by this sample meal plan, it's crucial to consume several small meals throughout the day. In fact, three meals and at least two snacks is ideal because consuming small, frequent meals throughout the day supports the stabilization of blood glucose levels much better than large, infrequent meals.

It's also crucial to eat close to the same time each day. The body likes routine and this is scientifically proven. The organs, such as the stomach, intestines, pancreas, and liver, have a natural daily rhythm. Organs synchronize with each other depending on food intake. Consuming food on a regular schedule enables these organs to function optimally and thus you will have improved glucose control.

A meal schedule is also important to prevent you from skipping meals. Skipping meals could lead to extreme hunger and thus you may be more inclined to consume a large meal full of carbs, especially if your blood sugar is low. A regular meal schedule will allow you to consume proper portions and you will likely be able to think more clearly and choose the right foods. Think about it—when you don't eat all day and finally come around to it, you're probably not thinking about eating something healthy, but instead you're thinking about eating something, *anything*. On the other hand, if you ate a balanced breakfast and lunch time comes four hours later, you will not be ravenous and will probably have no problem eating a carb-controlled dish.

Testing Blood Sugars

As mentioned, most practitioners will advise you to test your blood sugar four times per day: before breakfast and two hours after breakfast, lunch, and dinner. Your practitioner will also give you blood sugar goals such as the following:

- Before a meal (pre-prandial): 95 mg/dL or less

- Two hours after a meal (post-prandial): 120 mg/dL or less

Logging your meals and blood sugar readings in a chart is crucial. Your practitioner will likely give you a food and blood sugar log similar to the following:

Sample Meal/Blood Sugar Log

Date			
	Blood Sugar	Insulin Dose	Grams Carbs
Breakfast			
Snack			
Lunch			
Snack			
Dinner			
Snack			
Exercise			

Chapter Three

Physical Activity

Exercise is extremely beneficial for mother and baby during pregnancy, despite previous beliefs. You may have an older aunt or an elderly friend tell you "Don't overdo it" or "You need your rest." Some people still have the mindset that exercising during pregnancy can be dangerous. However, it's proven to have various advantages. In one randomized control trial regarding the efficacy of exercise in GDM management, 17 of 21 women in the exercise group (who were all insulin-dependent) were able to maintain normal glucose levels without using insulin! Another study found that women who engaged in diet plus exercise had lower glucose levels after six weeks of training than women who only followed a carb-controlled diet. This means a healthy diet and regular exercise can decrease your chance of needing insulin for glucose control.

Exercise has many positive effects on women with GDM. The benefits include easier labor, decreased back pain, improved muscle tone, decrease in constipation, increased energy levels, lower blood pressure, increased fetal oxygenation, normal baby birth weight, and easier postpartum weight loss.

Another very positive effect for women who exercise is improved mood, self-image, and psychological well-being. During pregnancy, you may not always feel that you are "glowing"; in fact, you may feel the complete opposite. There are days you'll feel a lack of confidence due to your growing and changing body. Exercise, whether it's a walk outdoors in the park or a quick indoor bike ride, can alleviate negative feelings and enhance your mood.[1]

Various types of exercises are safe during pregnancy, ranging from low-exerting exercises such as yoga to higher-exerting exercises such as jogging and aerobics. Of course, not all exercises are safe, including the following: recreational sports with increased risk of body injury (horseback riding, basketball, gymnastics), scuba diving, and exercising flat on your back after the second trimester (as it may obstruct inferior vena cava flow).

Your practitioner may advise you not to begin any new exercises and to continue with your regular exercise routine. While there are no specific guidelines for exercise, your practitioner will tell you their professional recommendations based on you as an individual, including your current and past health history.

There will be days you will be physically, and perhaps mentally, exhausted. However, take advantage of the days you have energy. Prioritize fitting exercise into your schedule, even if it is 15 to 20 minutes multiple times per week. Your body, your mind, and your baby will thank you.

The goal during pregnancy is not to run a marathon (though some women do) or to be your strongest and fittest self. The goals during pregnancy are to be as healthy as possible for you and baby, prevent health issues with nutrition and exercise, and, overall, have a smooth pregnancy and labor.

General exercise does not induce any harm on the fetus. The following exercises are great options to explore.

---

1   Cliantha Padayachee and Jeff S. Coombes. "Exercise Guidelines for Gestational Diabetes Mellitus," *World Journal of Diabetes* 6, no. 8 (2015): 1033-1044, doi: 10.4239/wjd.v6.i8.1033.

Walking. This is a highly recommended exercise for women with GDM. This full-body workout tones your muscles and is good for your heart. Additionally, as walking involves stretching, it can help alleviate aches and pains, such as in your hips, back, and legs. Also, walking after meals help you metabolize your food by pulling sugar out of the blood and into the cells (reducing blood sugar levels).

Yoga. This is one of the most beneficial prenatal exercises. Yoga allows you to focus on your breath and put you into a state of relaxation. Make no mistake, yoga is not a light workout—it can greatly strengthen your muscles, core, and stamina. Yoga is beneficial for those body parts that need extra attention during pregnancy, specifically your hips, pelvic floor, and overall posture.

Jogging. You may notice increased energy during the day and a better night's sleep with this type of exercise. If you were a runner prior to pregnancy, this may help you feel more like "yourself" in a time where your mind and body may feel so alien.

Aerobic dance. If you're feeling down, aerobic dance/Zumba is a great exercise to boost your mood. If you haven't been as social as before pregnancy, going to a dance class is a great way to socialize and get a full-body workout in. Aerobic dance allows you to get a good stretch in while toning your muscles.

Swimming. This is one of the best exercises to do when feeling the aches and pains associated with pregnancy. The buoyancy of the water allows you to feel weightless, taking some of the strain off of your joints. If you are in the later stages of pregnancy and are swelling often, water can help reduce it. If you have a planned water birth, moving your body and exercising in the water can allow you to better mentally prepare for the big day. Swimming is a very beneficial exercise, whether you are swimming laps or doing water aerobics.

Hiking. Hiking is a great exercise for maintaining strength and cardiovascular health. As a bonus, nature is a natural antidepressant. If you're feeling anxious or depressed, taking a hike may be just what you need. Nature has a restorative effect on many and can be a real mood-booster.

Rowing. This is a full-body workout that can also have a meditative effect. Whether you enjoy the sun beaming onto your face (increasing your vitamin D levels!) or the sound of the water gently splashing, this workout is low-impact and can help improve your balance.

Light- to moderate-strength training. Moms-to-be can greatly benefit from all that strength training has to offer. Strength training includes resistance machines, free weights, and bodyweight exercises. Upper-body exercises will greatly prepare you for all the lifting you'll be doing when baby comes. Back exercises can strengthen your muscles, alleviate lower back pain, and bring balance to the growing belly. Lower body exercises will allow you to better bear the weight of your pregnancy as your belly grows and keep your hips flexible.

Pelvic floor exercises. These exercises are known for reducing incontinence and poor bladder control postpartum, but they offer additional benefits. During pregnancy, a strong pelvic floor will help support your extra weight. After delivery, a strong pelvic floor will allow for better healing of your perineum due to extra blood circulation.

Resistance training. The Royal College of Obstetricians and Gynaecologists, the American College of Obstetrics and Gynecology, the Society of Obstetricians and Gynaecologists of Canada, and the Canadian Society for Exercise Physiology all recommend the use of resistance training for pregnant women; however, there are no specific guidelines yet provided.

Chapter Four

Recipes

Now that you're familiar with what GDM entails and the nutrition recommendations for keeping your blood sugar controlled, you can put all the pieces together by exploring the GDM-friendly recipes I've developed. Too many women are told how many carbs to eat and what foods to *avoid,* but are left unsure of exactly *what* to eat. Getting diagnosed with GDM does not mean you have to sacrifice flavor and taste with your food. Pregnancy is a special time where you should relax and enjoy yourself. For many, a big part of relaxation and joy involves food. These recipes will allow you to explore meals you might have never known you'd enjoy. These recipes will also allow you to indulge in all-time favorites, with a healthier spin that won't leave your blood sugar spiked. Many of the foods in the recipes were chosen with your baby kept in mind—foods that will provide key nutrients for optimal development, such as avocados, salmon, and veggies. I truly believe there is always a healthier alternative to foods, and after trying these recipes, I think you'll believe it, too.

The recipes include breakfast, lunch and dinner, snacks, and desserts. Each recipe includes the nutrition breakdown per serving, such as the calories; grams of fat, protein, and carbs; milligrams of sodium; and the carb counts, which will be useful when meal planning and complying with the recommended carb count as directed by your healthcare provider. For a refresher on the range of carbohydrates per carb count, you can refer to page 49. The sodium content is especially important if you have high blood pressure and are monitoring your sodium intake.

Please note that the optional choices are not included in the nutrition breakdown. Also, always check your individual food products labels, as nutrition information varies based on product.

Breakfast

Many women with GDM struggle with elevated blood sugar levels in the morning, despite the countless bedtime snacks they have alternated through in hopes of getting a normal fasted blood sugar reading. Starting your day with a balanced breakfast will help normalize your blood sugar throughout the rest of the day and set you up for success. While bagels, muffins, and other foods with refined carbs aren't in the recipe list, you will find a plethora of other high-fiber, no-added-sugar, nutrient-dense breakfasts that will energize and satiate you.

Balanced Yogurt Bowl

Yield: 1 serving | Prep time: 3 to 5 minutes

1 cup full-fat plain Greek yogurt

1 tablespoon chia seeds

¼ cup sliced strawberries

1 tablespoon slivered almonds

2 tablespoons toasted coconut flakes

Mix ingredients in bowl or layer ingredients as desired. Enjoy!

Nutrition: 413 calories, 23g total fat, 28g protein, 28g carbohydrates, 9g fiber, 109mg sodium

Carb count: **1½**

Simple Breakfast Porridge

Yield: 2 servings | Prep time: 3 minutes | Cook time: 10 minutes

1 cup rolled oats

ground cinnamon, to taste

2½ cups water, divided

1 tablespoon ground flaxseeds or chia seeds

Toppings (optional):

1 small apple, grated

banana, sliced

½ cup frozen or fresh berries

1. Place oats, cinnamon, and 2 cups of water in a small saucepan. Stir over low heat for 5 minutes. Let the oats simmer for about 5 minutes. Add the remaining water as needed until desired consistency is achieved.

2. Divide the porridge equally into 2 bowls. Stir in ground flaxseeds or chia seeds. Top with your optional choice of fruit.

Nutrition: 188 calories, 5g total fat, 6g protein, 34g carbohydrates, 9g fiber, 8mg sodium

Carb count: **2**

Ramekin Eggs

Yield: 2 (2-egg) servings | Prep time: 5 minutes | Cook time: 20 minutes

½ teaspoon butter, plus more as needed

1 large tomato, diced

1 large portobello mushroom, diced

¼ cup baby spinach leaves

4 eggs

1 ounce cheddar cheese, shredded

2 slices Ezekiel flax toast, to serve, optional

1. Preheat the oven to 400°F.

2. Grease four ramekins with the butter. You may use four sections of a muffin pan if you do not have ramekins.

3. Sauté the tomato and mushroom in a medium pan over medium heat until slightly browned, about four minutes. Then, add the spinach leaves. Stir for about 20 seconds and then remove from heat.

4. Spoon the tomato, mushroom, and spinach mixture into each ramekin. Crack an egg on top of each and add the shredded cheese.

5. Bake in oven for about 15 minutes.

6. Serve each portion with 1 slice of flax Ezekiel toast (buttered, if desired).

Nutrition: 223 calories, 15g total fat, 17g protein, 3g carbohydrates, 1g fiber, 245mg sodium

Carb count: **0**

Egg Muffins

Yield: 4 (3-muffin) servings | Prep time: 5 minutes | Cook time: 16 minutes

4 pieces cooked turkey bacon

6 eggs

2 ounces cheddar cheese

onion, tomato, or any other veggie toppings, optional

Ezekiel flax toast or side salad, optional

1. Preheat the oven to 400°F.

2. In a skillet over medium heat, scramble the eggs, about 4 minutes, and add to lightly greased 12-muffin pan.

3. Distribute the turkey bacon, cheese, and optional toppings into each muffin cup. Do not overfill, as the muffins will rise when cooking.

4. Bake for about 12 minutes or until egg is cooked through. While the muffins are baking, you may prepare the toast or side salad if desired.

Nutrition: 255 calories, 17g total fat, 23g protein, 1g carbohydrates, 0g fiber, 464mg sodium

Carb count: **0**

Veggie Frittata

Yield: 2 servings | Prep time: 5 minutes | Cook time: 25 minutes

1 tablespoon coconut oil

½ cup leeks, halved lengthwise, thinly sliced

½ red onion, finely chopped

¾ cup peeled and cubed small red potatoes

1 large zucchini, thinly sliced

4 eggs, lightly beaten

3 ounces cheddar cheese

black pepper, to taste

fresh or dried basil or cilantro, to taste

side salad, optional

1. Preheat the oven to 425°F.

2. Heat coconut oil over medium heat in a small skillet. Add leeks, onion, and potatoes. Lightly season with pepper and fresh or dried basil and cilantro.

3. Cook until leeks and onion are translucent, about 5 minutes.

4. Add zucchini, eggs, and cheese. Quickly stir to combine. Cook on medium heat for 2 to 3 minutes or until the edges become firm.

5. Transfer skillet to the oven and bake until egg is cooked through, 10 to 15 minutes..

6. Once done, flip onto a plate, cut into wedges, and serve with optional salad.

Nutrition: 503 calories, 33g total fat, 26g protein, 26g carbohydrates, 3g fiber, 538mg sodium

Carb count: **2**

Chia Seed French Toast

Yield: 2 (2-slice) servings | Prep time: 3 minutes | Cook time: 10 minutes

2 eggs, whisked

½ cup unsweetened vanilla almond milk (or milk of choice)

vanilla extract, to taste

1 teaspoon butter

4 slices Ezekiel flax bread

1 cup strawberries, fresh

ground cinnamon, to taste

½ teaspoon chia seeds, to top

1. In a large bowl, mix together eggs and milk. Add vanilla to mixture, to taste.

2. Heat butter in a large pan over medium heat.

3. Dip a slice of bread into the milk and egg mixture. Transfer to the pan. Cook each side until golden brown, 2 to 3 minutes. Repeat for each slice of bread.

4. Serve with sliced strawberries, cinnamon, and sprinkled chia seeds.

Nutrition: 264 calories, 9g total fat, 17g protein, 30g carbohydrates, 9g fiber, 273mg sodium

Carb count: **1½**

Avocado Toast with Egg

Yield: 2 servings | Prep time: 2 minutes | Cook time: 7 minutes

1 tablespoon butter

2 eggs

2 slices Ezekiel flax bread, toasted

1 avocado, halved

2 tomato slices

1 tablespoon chia seeds

1. Melt butter in a medium pan over medium heat. Add two eggs to the pan and cook over hard (or to your liking), about 4 minutes.

2. Place each avocado half on a piece of toasted bread. Mash with fork, then add cooked egg on top of avocado toast. Finally, top with a tomato slice.

3. Sprinkle ½ tablespoon of chia seeds over each piece.

Nutrition: 354 calories, 22g total fat, 15g protein, 19g carbohydrates, 7g fiber, 138mg sodium

Carb count: **1**

Low-Carb Pancakes

Yield: 3 (2-pancake) servings | Prep time: 5 minutes | Cook time: 10 to 15 minutes

1 cup almond flour

2 large eggs

¼ cup water

¼ teaspoon pink Himalayan salt

2 tablespoons coconut oil, divided

1 tablespoon maple syrup, to top

1. In a medium bowl, whisk together the almond flour, eggs, water, salt, and 1 tablespoon coconut oil. Let the batter sit for 2 minutes.

2. Add the remaining coconut oil to a nonstick pan over medium heat. Add a portion of batter to the skillet. Once bubbles appear, about 3 minutes, flip with a spatula and cook for another 2 to 3 minutes. Repeat with remaining batter.

3. Drizzle with maple syrup when finished.

Nutrition: 199 calories, 17g total fat, 6g protein, 7g carbohydrates, 1g fiber, 188mg sodium

Carb count: ½

Eggs Florentina

Yield: 2 servings | Prep time: 5 minutes | Cook time: 5 to 9 minutes

10 ounces chopped frozen or fresh spinach

1 tablespoon butter

4 medium eggs

2 tablespoons grated Parmesan cheese

1. If spinach is frozen, thaw it either in the microwave, counter, or a pan with water.

2. Heat the butter in pan over medium heat and then add the thawed spinach.

3. Heat the spinach for about 2 minutes. When the spinach is hot, crack the eggs on top. Cover the pan with a lid for another 2 minutes.

4. Take the lid off and sprinkle the cheese on top of the eggs. Replace lid on the pan and cook until the cheese is melted and eggs are cooked to your liking, for another 2 to 5 minutes.

Nutrition: 219 calories, 17g total fat, 15g protein, 2g carbohydrates, 0g fiber, 283mg sodium

Carb count: **0**

Flaxseed Meal Pudding

Yield: 1 serving | Prep time: 1 minute | Cook time: 2 minutes

¼ cup flaxseed meal

¼ cup water

1 large egg

½ packet stevia

1. Mix the flaxseed meal, water, and egg in a microwave-safe bowl.

2. Microwave on high for about 45 seconds. Mix. Microwave again for another 45 to 60 seconds.

3. Add ½ packet stevia to bowl to sweeten.

Nutrition: 196 calories, 17g total fat, 11g protein, 8g carbohydrates, 8g fiber, 80mg sodium

Carb count: **0**

Vanilla Chia Seed Pudding

Yield: 4 (½-cup) servings | Prep time: 10 minutes, plus 1 hour to refrigerate

½ cup heavy cream

1 cup full-fat coconut milk

⅛ teaspoon pink Himalayan salt

2 packets stevia

2 teaspoons vanilla extract

⅓ cup chia seeds

1. Mix all ingredients in a medium bowl.

2. Let sit for a few minutes and then stir again until mixed well.

3. Cover bowl and place in refrigerator until mixture is thick, similar to pudding consistency, about 1 hour.

Nutrition: 350 calories, 31g total fat, 5g protein, 14g carbohydrates, 7g fiber, 74mg sodium

Carb count: **½**

Breakfast BLT Salad

Yield: 2 servings | Prep time: 5 minutes | Cook time: 20 minutes

4 strips turkey bacon

3 cups shredded kale

1 teaspoon red wine vinegar

2 teaspoons extra-virgin olive oil

⅛ teaspoon pink Himalayan salt

1 avocado, sliced

10 grape tomatoes, halved

2 large eggs, hard boiled, chopped

black pepper, to taste, optional

1. Cook turkey bacon according to package instructions. When the bacon has finished cooking, chop into small pieces.

2. While turkey bacon is cooking, combine the kale, vinegar, olive oil, and salt in a large bowl. Massage with hands until kale softens.

3. Divide the kale mixture between two serving bowls. Top with bacon, sliced avocado, tomatoes, and egg.

Nutrition: 387 calories, 24g total fat, 26g protein, 22g carbohydrates, 10g fiber, 533mg sodium

Carb count: **1**

Apple Cinnamon Waffles

Yield: 8 (4-inch) waffles | Prep time: 3 minutes | Cook time: 24 minutes

1½ cups almond flour

½ cup flaxseed meal

1 scoop Garden of Life vanilla protein powder

1 tablespoon ground cinnamon

2 teaspoons baking powder

⅓ cup stevia, optional

4 large eggs

1 cup finely chopped apple

¾ cup unsweetened almond milk

¼ cup melted butter

1 teaspoon vanilla extract

1. Preheat waffle iron; grease, if necessary.

2. In a large bowl, whisk together the almond flour, flaxseed meal, protein powder, cinnamon, baking powder, and stevia, if using.

3. Stir in the eggs, apple, almond milk, butter, and vanilla extract. Mix until combined well.

4. Spoon batter into waffle iron and close lid. Cook until golden brown on each side, about 3 minutes per waffle.

5. Repeat with remaining batter.

Nutrition: 174 calories, 14g total fat, 8g protein, 7g carbohydrates, 4g fiber, 143mg sodium

Carb count: ½

Avocado Frittata

Yield: 6 servings | Prep time: 5 to 7 minutes | Cook time: 15 to 20 minutes

2 teaspoons avocado oil

8 eggs, whisked

½ cup grated mozzarella cheese

¼ cup sliced green onion

1 large avocado, halved, sliced lengthwise

2 ounces feta cheese

½ teaspoon Italian seasoning mix

1. Adjust the oven rack so it's 4 to 5 inches under the broiler. Turn broiler on to low.

2. Heat the oil in an oven-proof pan over medium-low heat. Add the eggs to the pan and cook for about 2 minutes.

3. Add the grated mozzarella and sliced green onion. Cook for 5 minutes or until the eggs look halfway done.

4. When eggs are halfway done, lay the avocado slices on top and sprinkle with the feta cheese and Italian seasoning mix.

5. Cover the pan with a lid and cook for another 3 minutes or until the eggs appear cooked through and the cheese is beginning to melt.

6. Remove the lid and place the frittata under the broiler. Cook for another 2 minutes. Carefully watch the dish to ensure it doesn't burn!

Nutrition: 202 calories, 15g total fat, 12g protein, 3g carbohydrates, 2g fiber, 248mg sodium

Carb count: **0**

Chocolate Banana Protein Pancakes

Yield: 3 (2-pancake) servings | Prep time: 5 minutes | Cook time: 6 minutes

2 scoops chocolate whey protein powder

2 tablespoons Bob's Red Mill pancake flour

2 tablespoons chia seeds

½ teaspoon baking powder

2 eggs, whisked

1 banana, mashed

4 tablespoons unsweetened almond milk

1 tablespoon butter

1. In a medium bowl, combine the protein powder, pancake flour, chia seeds, and baking powder together with a whisk.

2. In a separate bowl, combine the eggs, banana, and almond milk.

3. Pour the wet ingredients into the dry ingredients. Mix gently and be careful to not over-mix.

4. Heat butter in a large skillet over medium heat.

5. Pour a portion of the batter into the skillet. Once bubbles appear, about 3 minutes, flip with a spatula and cook for another 2 to 3 minutes.

Nutrition: 265 calories, 7g total fat, 19g protein, 23g carbohydrates, 9g fiber, 125mg sodium

Carb count: **1**

Cinnamon Hemp Hearts

Yield: 6 servings | Prep time: 1 minute | Cook time: 10 minutes

3½ cups unsweetened coconut milk

1 cup crushed pecans

½ cup hemp heart seeds

1½ teaspoons ground cinnamon

½ teaspoon vanilla extract

1 teaspoon maple syrup

¼ teaspoon allspice

stevia, to taste, optional

⅓ cup flaxseed meal

⅓ cup chia seeds

3 tablespoons butter

⅛ teaspoon psyllium husk, to thicken, optional

1. Heat coconut milk in a pot over medium heat.

2. Add pecans to a separate pan to toast over medium heat, about 4 minutes. Stir frequently to avoid burning.

3. Add hemp heart seeds, cinnamon, maple syrup, vanilla extract, and allspice, to the coconut milk and mix. Then, add stevia, if using, flaxseed meal, chia seeds, butter, and psyllium husk, if using. Mix well. Heat for about 6 minutes.

4. Once mixture is well heated, add the toasted pecans to pot and then serve.

Nutrition: 381 calories, 33g total fat, 10g protein, 18g carbohydrates, 14g fiber, 67mg sodium

Carb count: **1**

Bacon Avocado Breakfast "Burrito"

Yield: 2 servings | Prep time: 10 minutes | Cook time: 15 minutes

4 strips turkey bacon	1 cup romaine lettuce, chopped
2 eggs	1 Roma tomato, sliced
2 teaspoons butter, divided	½ large avocado, sliced
2 tablespoons mayonnaise	salt and black pepper, to taste

1. Cook turkey bacon according to package directions.

2. While turkey bacon is cooking, whisk eggs in a bowl. Season with salt and pepper to taste.

3. Heat a pan over medium heat. Melt 1 teaspoon of the butter in pan and add half of the egg mixture to create an "egg crepe" by spreading the egg thinly over the bottom of the pan. Cook for about 1 minute until ready to flip, then flip with spatula. When fully cooked, transfer to a plate.

4. Repeat with the remaining butter and egg mix.

5. Spread the mayonnaise on the crepes. Add lettuce, tomato, bacon, and avocado. Roll and enjoy as a burrito.

Nutrition: 341 calories, 27g total fat, 20g protein, 5g carbohydrates, 4g fiber, 599mg sodium

Carb count: **0**

Sweet Potato Fried Egg Bowl

Yield: 2 servings | Prep time: 10 minutes | Cook time: 15 minutes

4 pieces turkey bacon

1 tablespoon butter, divided

1 medium sweet potato, peeled and chopped into small cubes

2 eggs

1 tablespoon fresh chopped basil

black pepper, to taste

1. Cook turkey bacon according to package directions. When it is fully cooked, chop the bacon into small pieces.

2. Melt ½ tablespoon butter in a pan over medium-high heat. Add cubed sweet potato. Cook for approximately 10 minutes, until sweet potato is fork-tender.

3. While the sweet potato is cooking, heat remaining ½ tablespoon butter in another pan over medium-high heat. Cook the eggs over hard, or to your liking.

4. Once finished, divide the sweet potato between 2 plates. Top each with 1 egg, bacon pieces, and fresh basil. Season with black pepper, to taste.

Nutrition: 244 calories, 14g total fat, 20g protein, 12g carbohydrates, 2g fiber, 532mg sodium

Carb count: **1**

Portobello Veggie Stack

Yield: 2 servings | Prep time: 10 minutes | Cook time: 20 minutes

2 large portobello mushrooms

1 tablespoon butter

1 medium zucchini, halved and thinly sliced

1 red bell pepper, julienned

1 cup baby spinach

½ avocado

1 teaspoon dried basil

1 teaspoon fresh cilantro

2 tablespoons crumbled feta cheese

salt and black pepper, to taste

1. Preheat the oven to 350°F.

2. Sprinkle the mushrooms with salt and pepper, to taste. Bake for 20 minutes. Meanwhile, heat a pan over medium heat. Melt butter and sauté zucchini, bell pepper, and spinach to your liking.

3. Once the mushrooms are finished, place on serving dishes. Mash avocado onto each mushroom cap. Top with spinach, zucchini, and bell pepper. Lastly, sprinkle on basil, cilantro and feta cheese.

Nutrition: 207 calories, 13g total fat, 7g protein, 14g carbohydrates, 6g fiber, 233mg sodium

Carb count: **1**

Italian Eggs

Yield: 2 servings | Prep time: 5 minutes | Cook time: 5 to 7 minutes

½ cup natural marinara sauce

½ cup chopped spinach

4 eggs

¼ cup mozzarella cheese

1 teaspoon fresh basil

salt and black pepper, to taste

1. Add marinara sauce to a small unheated skillet.

2. Add the spinach and break in the eggs. Season with salt and pepper to taste, and then top with cheese. Place the skillet over medium-high heat.

3. Once the marinara sauce starts bubbling, reduce heat to medium-low. Cover and cook for 5 to 6 minutes, or until egg is cooked to your liking.

4. Top with fresh basil and serve.

Nutrition: 232 calories, 15g total fat, 17g protein, 5g carbohydrates, 1g fiber, 336mg sodium

Carb count: **0**

Cheesy Cauliflower Broccoli Tots

Yield: 3 servings | Prep time: 15 minutes | Cook time: 25 minutes

3 cups cauliflower florets

3 cups broccoli florets

1 cup shredded cheddar cheese

1 egg

salt and black pepper, to taste

1. Preheat the oven to 400°F.

2. Bring a pot of water to a boil. Add the cauliflower and broccoli florets and cook for 10 minutes.

3. Add the florets to a food processor. Process until fine, unless you desire a chunkier consistency. Once finished processing, remove extra moisture from cauliflower and broccoli.

4. Transfer to a large bowl. Add in the cheese and stir in the egg.

5. Roll mixture into tot shapes.

6. Place the tots on a baking sheet. Bake for about 25 minutes.

Nutrition: 246 calories, 17g total fat, 16g protein, 8g carbohydrates, 3g fiber, 349mg sodium

Carb count: ½

Breakfast Pizza Muffins

Yield: 8 muffins | Prep time: 10 minutes | Cook time: 35 minutes

4 thick chicken sausage links

6 eggs

½ cup heavy cream

1 teaspoon dried oregano

1 cup shredded mozzarella

1 cup pizza sauce

salt and black pepper, to taste

1. Preheat the oven to 325°F.

2. Cook chicken sausage according to package instructions, then slice the sausages into bite-sized pieces.

3. Mix the eggs, cream, salt and pepper, and oregano in a bowl.

4. Add the egg mixture to the muffin pan until each of 8 cups are filled a third of the way.

5. Divide the cheese evenly between each cup. Then, to each cup, add 1 tablespoon of pizza sauce, some of the cooked chicken sausage, and more of the egg mixture.

6. Bake for 20 to 25 minutes.

Nutrition: 219 calories, 16g total fat, 13g protein, 5g carbohydrates, 1g fiber, 554mg sodium

Carb count: **0**

Peanut Butter Muffin

Yield: 1 serving | Prep time: 1 to 2 minutes | Cook time: 1 minute in microwave (or 10 to 12 minutes in oven)

butter, as needed

1 large egg

2 teaspoons coconut flour

2 teaspoons peanut butter

pinch baking soda

pinch salt

1. Grease a ramekin with butter.

2. In a mug, mix all the ingredients together with a fork until the mixture is lump-free.

3. Place the mixture into the greased ramekin. Cook in the microwave on high for 1 minute, or bake in oven at 400°F for 10 to 12 minutes.

Nutrition: 195 calories, 14g total fat, 9g protein, 5g carbohydrates, 2g fiber, 237mg sodium

Carb count: **0**

Spinach & Mozzarella Muffin

Yield: 1 serving | Prep time: 1 to 2 minutes | Cook time: 1 minute in microwave (or 10 to 12 minutes in oven)

butter, as needed

1 large egg

2 teaspoons coconut flour

2 tablespoons shredded mozzarella cheese

1 tablespoon chopped fresh baby spinach leaves

pinch baking soda

pinch salt

1. Grease a ramekin with butter.

2. In a mug, mix all the ingredients together with a fork until the mixture is lump-free.

3. Place the mixture into the greased ramekin. Cook in the microwave on high for 1 minute or bake in oven at 400°F for 10 to 12 minutes.

Nutrition: 170 calories, 12g total fat, 11g protein, 4g carbohydrates, 2g fiber, 298mg sodium

Carb count: **0**

4-Ingredient Cottage Cheese Pancakes

Yield: 2 (2-pancake) servings | Prep time: 3 minutes | Cook time: 5 to 6 minutes

½ cup cottage cheese

½ cup rolled oats

3 eggs

1 teaspoon chia seeds

1 teaspoon butter, to grease pan

1. Mix the cottage cheese, rolled oats, eggs, and chia seeds in a bowl until smooth.

2. Melt the butter in a pan over medium heat.

3. Add a portion of the batter to pan. Once bubbles appear, flip with a spatula. Cook until both sides are golden brown, 5 to 6 minutes total. Repeat with remaining batter.

Nutrition: 245 calories, 11g total fat, 19g protein, 16g carbohydrates, 2g fiber, 354mg sodium

Carb count: **1**

Lunch/Dinner

Your GDM diagnosis doesn't have to be crippling. Take it as an opportunity to evaluate your usual dietary intake and establish good habits that you can carry on postpartum. This is your chance to learn about and change your overall approach to nutrition. With these lunch and dinner recipes, you may find yourself feeling less sluggish, full longer, and completely satisfied. That's because these recipes don't ask you to sacrifice flavor for health. From soups to salads to stir-fries to one-pan bakes, you will explore a variety of low-carb dishes that contain good amounts of fiber, protein, and healthy fats. You'll find that many of the lunches and dinners contain veggies that come in all different colors and textures. So, go on and explore what these recipes have to offer.

Colorful Tuna Salad

Yield: 3 servings | Prep time: 10 minutes

1 cup mixed greens

1 cup cherry tomatoes, halved

½ cup pitted black olives

½ cup sliced button mushrooms

1 (5-ounce) can tuna, drained

1 tablespoon small capers

2 eggs, hard boiled, peeled, quartered

1 tablespoon olive oil

1 tablespoon red wine vinegar

Place mixed greens, tomatoes, olives, mushrooms, tuna, capers, and eggs into a bowl. Mix. Add olive oil and vinegar, and mix again. Divide equally between 3 bowls.

Nutrition: 178 calories, 13g total fat, 7g protein, 12g carbohydrates, 4g fiber, 491mg sodium

Carb count: **1**

Spicy Sweet Potato Soup

Yield: 4 servings | Prep time: 10 minutes | Cook time: 25 minutes

1 tablespoon olive oil

1 large onion, roughly chopped

2 cloves garlic, crushed

1 teaspoon red curry paste (mild or spicy)

1½ pounds sweet potatoes, peeled, diced

2 cups low-sodium vegetable stock

1 cup coconut milk

½ cup fresh chopped cilantro

½ cup fresh chopped basil

1 lime, quartered

4 tablespoons pumpkin seeds

side salad, optional

1. Heat olive oil in a saucepan over medium-low heat. Add onion and garlic; cook until onions turn translucent, about 3 minutes. Add curry paste and stir. Cook for about 1 minute.

2. Add sweet potatoes and broth. If potatoes are not fully covered, add water or more broth. Cover saucepan with lid and bring to a boil.

3. Lower heat and simmer for about 20 minutes, until sweet potato is soft.

4. Once the soup has cooled, blend. Slowly stir in coconut milk to control consistency.

5. Divide soup into four bowls. Top each serving with cilantro, basil, lime, and pumpkin seeds. Serve with side salad, if desired.

Nutrition: 195 calories, 7g total fat, 8g protein, 28.5g carbohydrates, 5g fiber, 100mg sodium

Carb count: **2**

Salmon Miso Soup

Yield: 3 servings | Prep time: 10 minutes | Cook time: 15 minutes

4 cups water

4 tablespoons miso paste

2 teaspoons grated ginger

2 (4-ounce) salmon fillets

½ head broccoli, cut into florets

½ bunch asparagus, cut into ½-inch pieces

6 button mushrooms, thinly sliced

2 shallots, thinly sliced

1 cup cooked quinoa

2 teaspoons sesame oil

2 teaspoons low-sodium soy sauce

2 tablespoons sesame seeds, toasted

1 sheet nori (seaweed) paper, thinly cut with scissors

1. In a saucepan over medium heat, combine 4 cups of water with miso paste and ginger. Add salmon filets, cover with lid, and poach over medium-low heat for 5 to 8 minutes until the salmon is mostly cooked through.

2. Add broccoli, asparagus, mushrooms, and shallots. Cook covered over low heat for about 4 to 5 minutes or until vegetables begin to soften.

3. Divide cooked quinoa between three bowls, then place the salmon over the quinoa. Then, equally divide the soup over the salmon.

4. Drizzle each bowl with sesame oil, soy sauce, sesame seeds, and nori paper.

Nutrition: 269 calories, 10g total fat, 25g protein, 27g carbohydrates, 5g fiber, 542mg sodium

Carb count: **1½**

Cauliflower Leek Soup

Yield: 5 servings | Prep time: 10 minutes | Cook time: 30 minutes

2 tablespoons olive oil

1½ leeks, sliced

1 large fennel bulb, sliced

2 small heads of cauliflower, cut into florets

¾ pound potatoes, peeled, diced

4 cups low-sodium vegetable broth

2 bay leaves

1 teaspoon dried tarragon

1 teaspoon caraway seeds

6 teaspoons sliced chives

1. Heat the oil in a large saucepan over low heat. Add the leeks and fennel. Stir well. Cover and cook on low heat for about 10 minutes or until ingredients have softened.

2. Add the cauliflower and potatoes to the pan. Cook for 5 minutes.

3. Pour in the broth. Add the bay leaves, tarragon, and caraway seeds. Bring to a boil. Partially cover with lid and simmer for about 15 minutes, or until the potatoes are fork-tender. Remove from heat. Scoop out the vegetables and set aside about 1½ cups of liquid.

4. Let the vegetables cool, then blend well. If the soup is too thick, add liquid that was set aside in increments.

5. To serve, divide the soup evenly into 5 bowls and top with chives.

Nutrition: 180 calories, 7g total fat, 7g protein, 28g carbohydrates, 6g fiber, 140mg sodium

Carb count: **1½**

Slow-Cooker Beef Teriyaki Lettuce Wraps

Yield: 6 servings | Prep time: 10 minutes | Cook time: 6½ to 9½ hours

1 small onion, diced

3 cloves garlic, minced

½ cup honey

½ cup low-sodium soy sauce

⅓ cup rice wine vinegar

1 teaspoon ground ginger

2 pounds beef (boneless eye of round roast), halved lengthwise

⅓ cup water

2 heaping tablespoons arrowroot powder

12 large romaine lettuce leaves

4 scallions, chopped

1. In a medium bowl, combine onion, garlic, honey, soy sauce, rice wine vinegar, and ginger. Combine well.

2. Place beef in slow cooker and cover with soy sauce mixture.

3. Cover and cook on high for 6 to 7 hours or low for 8 to 9 hours.

4. Remove beef from slow cooker and place on a large cutting board. Leave remaining mixture in the slow cooker.

5. In a small bowl, combine water and arrowroot powder. Pour into mixture in the slow cooker. Stir to combine. Cover and heat on high for 20 to 30 minutes to thicken sauce. Meanwhile, shred the beef using 2 forks.

6. Once sauce has finished thickening, turn off the slow cooker. Add beef back to slow cooker and stir to cover in sauce.

7. Equally divide on top of lettuce leaves. Garnish with scallions.

Nutrition: 390 calories, 14g total fat, 34g protein, 32g carbohydrates, 2g fiber, 693mg sodium

Carb count: **2**

Beef and Chicken Sausage Empanadas

Yield: 6 (2-empanada) servings | Prep time: 7 to 10 minutes | Cook time: 20 to 25 minutes

For the filling:

8 ounces ground grass-fed beef

8 ounces chicken sausage, casings removed

½ cup onion, diced

2 cloves garlic, minced

2 tablespoons tomato paste

3 green onions, chopped

8 green olives, chopped

salt and black pepper, to taste

For the dough:

1½ cups shredded mozzarella cheese

3 tablespoons cream cheese

¾ cup almond flour

1 large egg

1 teaspoon garlic powder

1 teaspoon onion powder

1 teaspoon Italian seasoning

1 teaspoon pink Himalayan salt

½ teaspoon black pepper

1. To make the filling, add the ground beef, chicken sausage, onion, garlic, salt, and pepper to a large skillet. Sauté over medium heat until the meat is cooked through, about 15 minutes.

2. Drain excess grease. Mix in the tomato paste and sauté for 5 minutes.

3. Transfer mixture to a bowl. Add green onions and olives and season with salt and pepper, to taste. Set aside.

4. To make the dough, in a large mixing bowl, combine the mozzarella cheese and cream cheese. Microwave for 1 minute. Stir, then microwave for 1 more minute.

5. Mix in almond flour, egg, garlic powder, onion powder, Italian seasoning, salt, and pepper. Mix until well combined.

6. To prepare the empanadas, preheat the oven to 425°F. Line 2 baking sheets with parchment paper; grease, if desired.

7. Spread the dough out in a thin, even layer across 1 baking sheet. Use the rim of a large drinking glass to cut circles in the dough. Place the circles onto the other baking sheet. Repeat until you have 12 circles.

8. Evenly divide the filling between the circles of dough. Fold the dough over and press the edges together with a fork.

9. Bake for 12 minutes or until golden brown.

Nutrition: 271 calories, 17g total fat, 22g protein, 6g carbohydrates, 1g fiber, 240mg sodium

Carb count: ½

Fast Baked Salmon

Yield: 2 servings | Prep time: 7 minutes | Cook time: 12 to 15 minutes

2 (4-ounce) salmon fillets

1 tablespoon avocado oil

pinch pink Himalayan salt

pinch black pepper

1 teaspoon dried basil

8 asparagus spears

4 slices onion

4 slices lemon

1 teaspoon fresh chopped parsley

1. Preheat the oven to 400°F.

2. In a medium bowl, season the salmon with avocado oil, salt, pepper, and dried basil.

3. Cut two sheets of foil large enough to wrap around the salmon and the asparagus.

4. Place 4 spears of asparagus on one sheet of foil. Layer a fillet of salmon over the asparagus. Top with 2 onion slices and 2 lemon slices. Wrap foil around salmon so it's completely enclosed. Repeat process with the second fillet of salmon.

5. Place both foil packets on a baking sheet. Bake for about 12 to 15 minutes.

6. Once salmon is cooked to your liking, transfer with a spatula to dish. Enjoy.

Nutrition: 331 calories, 23g total fat, 25g protein, 7g carbohydrates, 2g fiber, 54mg sodium

Carb count: ½

Noodle-less Lasagna

Yield: 12 servings | Prep time: 20 minutes | Cook time: 70 minutes

1½ pounds zucchini, thinly sliced lengthwise

1 pound ground beef

2 cups low-sugar pasta sauce

3 tablespoons Italian seasoning

1 pound ricotta cheese

8 ounces grated mozzarella cheese, plus more to top

½ cup grated Parmesan cheese

2 eggs

salt and black pepper, to taste

1. Place zucchini on greased baking sheet and bake at 400°F until slightly browned and tender (about 10 minutes). Once done, reduce oven temperature to 350°F.

2. While zucchini is baking, brown meat in a large skillet for 8 to 10 minutes. Once almost cooked through, add pasta sauce, Italian seasoning, salt, and pepper. Once finished, turn off heat and set aside.

3. In a separate bowl, mix ricotta with eggs, mozzarella, and Parmesan. Set aside.

4. When zucchini is done baking, remove from oven. Layer the bottom of a large baking dish with the meat and sauce mixture. Add zucchini strips followed by cheese and egg mixture. Layer until all ingredients are used up.

5. Place the dish in the oven at 350°F for 45 to 60 minutes, until egg and ricotta mixture is firm.

6. If adding additional mozzarella to melt on top of zucchini lasagna, add it 5 minutes before finished.

Nutrition: 325 calories, 21g total fat, 28g protein, 7g carbohydrates, 1g fiber, 589mg sodium

Carb count: ½

Thai Basil Chicken

Yield: 4 servings | Prep time: 2 minutes | Cook time: 11 minutes

2 tablespoons avocado oil

3 cloves fresh garlic, chopped

1 teaspoon fresh minced ginger

2 tablespoons fresh minced chiles

20 ounces boneless, skinless chicken breast, diced

1 tablespoon fish sauce

¼ cup fresh, roughly chopped basil

1 cup steamed broccoli or ½ cup brown rice, optional

1. Heat the avocado oil in a pan over medium heat. Add garlic, ginger, and chiles. Cook for 2 minutes or until sizzling.

2. Add the chicken to the pan. Cook for about 7 minutes, or until golden brown and cooked through.

3. Add the fish sauce and fresh basil. Stir and cook until the chicken is coated and the basil is wilted (about 2 minutes).

4. Remove from pan. Optionally, serve with 1 cup steamed broccoli or ½ cup brown rice per person.

Nutrition: 222 calories, 11g total fat, 28g protein, 2g carbohydrates, 0g fiber, 486mg sodium

Carb count: **0**

Poached Eggs over Chicken Sausage

Yield: 1 serving | Prep time: 3 minutes | Cook time: 10 minutes

2 links chicken sausage

1 tablespoon white wine vinegar

2 large eggs

¼ teaspoon coconut oil

1 tablespoon chopped onion or shallot

1 cup fresh baby spinach

pinch paprika

pinch red pepper flakes

1. Cook the chicken sausage according to package directions.

2. While the chicken sausage is cooking, fill a shallow pan with 1½ to 2 inches of water and bring to a boil. Once boiling, reduce to a low simmer and add the white wine vinegar. Crack the eggs into a small bowl and gently slide them into the water.

3. In a separate skillet, heat the coconut oil over medium heat. Sauté chopped onion for about 2 minutes, then remove from heat. Add spinach to the skillet with the onion. Cook until wilted, about 1 minute.

4. Once the eggs are done cooking (about 3 minutes), gently remove them with a spoon onto a dish.

5. Plate in the following order: onions and spinach, chicken sausage, and poached eggs. Top with a pinch of paprika and red pepper flakes.

Nutrition: 263 calories, 16g total fat, 25g protein, 4g carbohydrates, 1g fiber, 499mg sodium

Carb count: **0**

Caprese Balsamic Chicken

Yield: 4 servings | Prep time: 5 minutes | Cook time: 20 to 25 minutes

3 tablespoons avocado oil

1¼ pounds chicken breast

2 garlic cloves, minced

1 cup low-sodium chicken broth

½ cup balsamic vinegar

2 tablespoons roughly chopped fresh basil

4 ounces mozzarella cheese, sliced

1 Roma tomato, sliced

black pepper, to taste

1. Preheat broiler to high.

2. Thinly slice the chicken breasts. Heat oil in skillet on medium-high. Add chicken and brown on both sides, about 7 minutes. Reduce heat to medium-low and add garlic. Cook until garlic is tender, about 2 minutes; be sure not to burn it.

3. Add chicken broth and balsamic vinegar to the skillet. Turn heat back up to medium-high. Cover and simmer for about 10 minutes until chicken is cooked through.

4. Line a baking sheet with parchment paper. Place each chicken piece on baking sheet. Evenly divide the basil, mozzarella, and tomato slices between chicken. Broil until cheese is melted. Top with black pepper and serve.

Nutrition: 311 calories, 16g total fat, 34g protein, 6g carbohydrates, 1g fiber, 367mg sodium

Carb count: ½

Curried Salmon Cakes

Yield: 2 servings | Prep time: 3 minutes | Cook time: 8 minutes

1 (6-ounce) can salmon

½ cup finely chopped baby spinach

½ medium zucchini, grated

1 tablespoon curry powder

1 teaspoon red pepper flakes

1 teaspoon ground ginger

1 large egg

1 tablespoon butter

1. In a large bowl, combine the salmon, spinach, zucchini, curry powder, red pepper flakes, and ginger. Mix well. Add the egg; stir until combined.

2. Heat butter over medium heat in a skillet. While heating, form two salmons into patties. Add the patties to the skillet and cook each side until golden brown, about 4 minutes per side.

Nutrition: 231 calories, 13g total fat, 21g protein, 5g carbohydrates, 3g fiber, 384mg sodium

Carb count: **0**

Greek Salad Wrap

Yield: 6 servings | Prep time: 5 minutes | Cook time: 2 minutes

⅓ cup red wine vinegar

¼ cup extra-virgin olive oil

2 tablespoons finely chopped, fresh oregano

¼ teaspoon black pepper

8 cups chopped romaine lettuce

1½ cups cucumber, halved and sliced

1 cup grape tomatoes, halved

¼ cup pitted olives

¼ cup chopped red onion

1 package Ezekiel sprouted-grain tortillas

1. In a large bowl, mix vinegar, oil, oregano, and pepper. Add romaine lettuce, cucumber, tomatoes, olives, and onion, and toss to coat.

2. If desired, heat 6 tortillas in a pan or in an oven to desired crispiness.

3. Place 1½ cups of the salad mixture onto each wrap.

Nutrition: 328 calories, 22g total fat, 7g protein, 27g carbohydrates, 6g fiber, 145mg sodium

Carb count: **1½**

Tofu Lettuce Wrap with Peanut Sauce

Yield: 3 (3-wrap) servings | Prep time: 10 minutes | Cook time: 20 minutes

For the tofu mixture:

1 tablespoon avocado oil

1 cup firm tofu, crumbled

2 tablespoons cashew nuts

1 tablespoon red chili flakes

small handful fresh basil

1 tablespoon lime juice

1 tablespoon low-sodium soy sauce

For the peanut sauce:

1 tablespoon sweet chili sauce

1 tablespoon natural peanut butter

2 tablespoons water

For the wrap:

⅓ cup uncooked brown rice

9 large romaine leaves

1. Cook rice according to box directions.

2. Heat the oil over medium heat in a skillet. Add the crumbled tofu and cook for about 7 minutes, until crispy.

3. While the tofu is cooking, add the cashews, chili flakes, and fresh basil to a food processor. Process to crumb consistency.

4. Once tofu is crispy, add the cashew mixture to the skillet. Add lime juice and soy sauce. Cook on medium-low heat for another 5 minutes.

5. Add to the processor the sweet chili sauce, peanut butter, and water to make the peanut sauce. Adjust the consistency to your liking with more water.

6. Divide the cooked rice, tofu mixture, and peanut sauce drizzle between lettuce leaves.

Nutrition: 233 calories, 10g total fat, 8g protein, 24g carbohydrates, 3g fiber, 284mg sodium

Carb count: **1½**

Keep-It-Simple Beef Stew

Yield: 4 servings | Prep time: 10 minutes | Cook time: 8 hours

1 cup quartered small red potatoes

4 medium carrots, halved

1 small red onion, diced

1 pound beef stew meat

1 (10.75-ounce) can low-sodium cream of mushroom soup

1 cup low-sodium beef broth

½ teaspoon roughly chopped dried thyme

1 (10-ounce) package frozen cut green beans, thawed

1. In a 4-quart slow cooker, add potatoes, carrots, onion, stew meat, mushroom soup, beef broth, and thyme. Stir to combine.

2. Cover and cook on low heat for 8 hours. At 7 hours and 45 minutes, add thawed green beans and turn to high-heat setting. Cover and cook for 15 more minutes.

Nutrition: 273 calories, 7g total fat, 28g protein, 21g carbohydrates, 5g fiber, 188mg sodium

Carb count: **1**

Peanut Butter & Fig Crisps

Yield: 1 serving | Prep time: 3 minutes | Cook time: 0 minutes

2 GG Scandinavian Fiber Crispbread crackers

2 tablespoons natural peanut butter

2 dried figs, sliced

1 tablespoon pepitas

1 teaspoon coconut flakes

Top each crispbread with 1 tablespoon peanut butter, half the fig slices, ½ tablespoon pepitas, and ½ teaspoon coconut flakes.

Nutrition: 348 calories, 21g total fat, 11g protein, 32g carbohydrates, 12g fiber, 162mg sodium

Carb count: **2**

10-Minute Portobello Pizza

Yield: 3 (2-pizza) servings | Prep time: 6 minutes | Cook time: 6 to 8 minutes

2 tablespoons extra-virgin olive oil

2 teaspoons minced garlic

6 teaspoons Italian seasoning, divided

6 portobello mushrooms caps, stems removed

¾ cup low-sodium pizza sauce

1½ cups low-sodium mozzarella cheese

6 grape tomatoes, thinly sliced

red pepper flakes, to taste

1. Preheat the oven to a high broil and position the rack in the middle of the oven.

2. In a small bowl, combine the oil, garlic, and 4 teaspoons of Italian seasoning together.

3. Brush the bottoms of each mushroom with the garlic and oil mixture. Place each mushroom, oil side down, on a baking tray.

4. Top each mushroom with the pizza sauce, mozzarella cheese, and tomato slices, divided evenly. Broil for about 6 to 8 minutes, until cheese is melted.

5. Once finished cooking, sprinkle with the remaining Italian seasoning and red pepper flakes.

Nutrition: 349 calories, 22g total fat, 22g protein, 18g carbohydrates, 5g fiber, 489mg sodium

Carb count: **1**

Cauliflower Fried Rice

Yield: 4 servings | Prep time: 8 minutes | Cook time: 12 minutes

1 medium cauliflower head	2 eggs, beaten
2 tablespoons sesame oil, divided	3 tablespoons low-sodium soy sauce
1 large carrot, cubed	6 green onions, minced
2 garlic cloves, minced	4 tablespoons sesame seeds
1 cup frozen edamame	

1. Process cauliflower in food processor until it reaches a rice consistency.

2. Heat 1 tablespoon of sesame oil in a large skillet over medium heat. Add the carrot and garlic; stir fry until garlic is fragrant, about 4 minutes. Add the cauliflower, edamame, and remaining sesame oil. Stir fry for 4 minutes until the cauliflower is soft, but not mushy.

3. Before cauliflower gets mushy, make a well in the middle of the pan and reduce heat to low. Add the eggs. Stir gently until eggs are fully cooked, about 3 minutes.

4. Stir in the soy sauce and green onions for 1 minute.

5. Top with sesame seeds, 1 tablespoon per plate.

Nutrition: 257 calories, 15g total fat, 13g protein, 19g carbohydrates, 8g fiber, 540mg sodium

Carb count: **1**

One-Pan Pesto Chicken

Yield: 3 servings | Prep time: 10 minutes | Cook time: 20 minutes

2 tablespoons olive oil, divided

1 cup fresh basil

¼ cup grated Parmesan cheese

1 clove garlic, minced

½ teaspoon black pepper

1 pound chicken thighs, boneless and skinless

1 package mushrooms, halved

1 package cherry tomatoes

½ head broccoli, cut into florets

1 small zucchini, cut into thick slices

1. Preheat the oven to 400°F.

2. Make the pesto. In a food processor, process 1 tablespoons of olive oil, basil, Parmesan cheese, garlic, and pepper until smooth. Add water to adjust to preferred consistency.

3. To a large baking pan, add the chicken and mushrooms. Toss with the remaining tablespoon of olive oil and 2 tablespoons pesto. Bake for 10 minutes. Remove from oven and drain excess liquid.

4. Add the remaining vegetables and 2 tablespoons pesto. Toss to combine. Bake for an additional 10 minutes, or until chicken is cooked through.

Nutrition: 337 calories, 18g total fat, 30g protein, 11g carbohydrates, 3g fiber, 575mg sodium

Carb count: **1**

Ground Turkey Stir-Fry

Yield: 3 servings | Prep time: 10 minutes | Cook time: 10 minutes

1 tablespoon avocado oil

1 pound ground turkey

2 cloves garlic, minced

1 tablespoon grated ginger

1 bag rainbow salad (if you don't see this specifically, look for a bag of pre-chopped veggies containing a variation such as cauliflower, broccoli, carrots, and cabbage)

⅛ cup low-sodium soy sauce

4 scallions, sliced

1 tablespoon sesame seed oil

1. Heat avocado oil in large skillet over medium heat.

2. Add ground turkey to pan. Break up with a spoon and stir-fry until almost cooked through, about 7 minutes. Stir in garlic and ginger, then add rainbow salad vegetables and soy sauce. Stir-fry vegetables for an additional 3 minutes, or to desired consistency. Ensure turkey is cooked through.

3. Add sliced scallions and sesame seed oil to mixture. Stir quickly then remove from heat.

Nutrition: 360 calories, 20g total fat, 34g protein, 13g carbohydrates, 3g fiber, 463mg sodium

Carb count: **1**

Homemade Chicken & Vegetable Teriyaki

Yield: 4 servings | Prep time: 10 minutes | Cook time: 17 to 19 minutes

1 bag frozen Asian vegetables

1 tablespoon avocado oil

1 pound chicken breast, cubed

4 tablespoons coconut flour

1¼ cups water, divided

¼ cup low-sodium soy sauce

¼ cup maple syrup

1 tablespoon minced garlic

1 teaspoon fresh grated ginger

4 tablespoons scallions, sliced

4 tablespoons sesame seeds

1. Cook frozen vegetables according to package directions.

2. Heat avocado oil in large skillet over medium heat. Add chicken and cook for about 12 minutes or until inside is no longer pink.

3. While chicken is cooking, in a small bowl mix together flour and ¼ cup water. Set aside.

4. To make the teriyaki sauce, heat a small pot over medium-high heat. Add remaining water, soy sauce, maple syrup, garlic, and ginger. Stir. When it begins to bubble, add in flour mixture. Stir continuously for 5 to 7 minutes. Remove from heat and set aside until chicken is ready.

5. Once chicken is almost finished, add teriyaki sauce and cooked mixed vegetables. Stir to combine.

6. Divide chicken teriyaki evenly among 4 plates. Garnish each dish with scallions and sesame seeds.

Nutrition: 329 calories, 11g total fat, 30g protein, 26g carbohydrates, 5g fiber, 599mg sodium

Carb count: **1½**

Classic Pressure-Cooker Chicken Noodle Soup

Yield: 4 servings | Prep time: 10 minutes | Cook time: 20 minutes

3 tablespoons avocado oil

1 cup diced onion

2 cloves garlic

2 large chicken breasts, cubed

1 cup diced carrots

1 cup diced celery

½ (4-ounce) box Banza Chickpea Rotini, uncooked

8 cups low-sodium chicken broth

¼ teaspoon black pepper

1 cup frozen cooked peas

handful fresh parsley, roughly chopped

1. Put pressure cooker on high-heat setting. Once ready, add the avocado oil and chopped onion. Stir-fry until browned, about 3 minutes. Add garlic and chicken. Stir-fry until chicken begins to whiten on all sides, about 7 minutes.

2. Add diced carrots and celery, uncooked pasta, chicken broth, and pepper.

3. Pressure cook for about 10 minutes (it may take a few minutes to reach the pressure cooking point, extending the total cooking time). After 10 minutes, release pressure. Open and add frozen cooked peas (they will defrost in the heat and cool down soup).

4. Serve immediately with fresh chopped parsley.

Nutrition: 320 calories, 7g total fat, 39g protein, 32g carbohydrates, 8g fiber, 453mg sodium

Carb count: **2**

Nachos-in-a-Pepper

Yield: 5 servings | Prep time: 5 minutes | Cook time: 15 to 20 minutes

1 tablespoon chili powder

1 teaspoon ground cumin

1 teaspoon garlic powder

1 teaspoon paprika

½ teaspoon pink Himalayan salt

½ teaspoon black pepper

½ teaspoon oregano

¼ teaspoon red pepper flakes

1 pound ground beef

1 pound mini peppers, halved and seeded

1½ cups shredded cheddar cheese

½ cup chopped tomato

Toppings (optional):

sour cream

olives

jalapeno

cilantro

avocado

1. Preheat the oven to 400°F.

2. In a small bowl, combine the chili powder, cumin, garlic powder, paprika, salt, pepper, oregano, and red pepper flakes.

3. In a large skillet over medium heat, add ground beef. Break up clumps with a wooden spoon and brown until just cooked through, about 10 minutes. Add spice mixture and mix until well combined. Remove from heat.

4. Line a baking tray with parchment paper. Arrange mini peppers in a single layer with the cut-side facing up. Add ground beef mixture and shredded cheese. Bake 5 to 10 minutes, until cheese is melted.

5. Remove from oven. Top with chopped tomatoes and optional toppings.

Nutrition: 362 calories, 24g total fat, 31g protein, 8g carbohydrates, 2g fiber, 569mg sodium

Carb count: ½

Taco Salad

Yield: 5 servings | Prep time: 15 minutes | Cook time: 8 minutes

For the taco salad:

1 pound extra-lean ground beef

1 teaspoon ground cumin

1 teaspoon paprika

1 teaspoon chili powder

1 teaspoon garlic powder

¼ medium red onion, diced

½ cup shredded Mexican cheese

1 avocado, diced

½ cup halved cherry tomatoes

1 small romaine lettuce head, roughly chopped

For the avocado cilantro dressing:

1 small avocado

1 cup cilantro

¼ cup fresh lime juice

¼ teaspoon pink Himalayan salt

¼ teaspoon ground cumin

⅓ cup extra-virgin olive oil

2 to 4 tablespoons water, depending on preferred consistency

1. Heat a skillet over medium-high heat. Add beef and spices. Break up the meat with a wooden spoon. Stir and cook for about 7 minutes, or until the meat is cooked through.

2. While the meat is cooking, add the onion, cheese, avocado, tomatoes, and romaine lettuce to a large bowl.

3. Prepare the salad dressing: In a food processor, combine the avocado, cilantro, lime juice, pink Himalayan salt, cumin, and olive oil. Blend until smooth. Add water to adjust consistency

4. Once the meat is cooked through, sprinkle it over the salad. Add dressing and toss all ingredients.

Nutrition: 446 calories, 33g total fat, 29g protein, 11g carbohydrates, 7g fiber, 244mg sodium

Carb count: ½

Mini Pepper Tuna Melt

Yield: 2 (4-pepper) servings | Prep time: 7 minutes | Cook time: 5 minutes

1 (5-ounce) can tuna, drained

3½ tablespoons avocado oil mayonnaise

1 lemon, juiced

½ teaspoon black pepper

8 mini peppers, seeded and halved, stems on

2 ounces grated cheddar cheese

1. Preheat the oven to 350°F.

2. Line a baking sheet with parchment paper.

3. In a medium bowl, combine the tuna, mayo, lemon, and pepper. Mix well.

4. Divide the tuna among the mini pepper halves. Top with cheddar cheese.

5. Bake for 5 minutes or until cheese is melted.

Nutrition: 393 calories, 30g total fat, 22g protein, 9g carbohydrates, 2g fiber, 567mg sodium

Carb count: ½

Slightly Stuffed Jalapeno Baked Chicken

Yield: 4 servings | Prep time: 8 minutes | Cook time: 30 minutes

4 (5-ounce) chicken breasts

1 tablespoon olive oil

½ teaspoon paprika

¼ teaspoon pink Himalayan salt

4 ounces cream cheese

1 cup grated cheddar cheese

4 jalapenos, de-seeded, finely diced

1. Preheat the oven to 375°F. Line a baking sheet with parchment paper.

2. Place the chicken breasts on the parchment paper. Cut about 7 slits widthwise into each chicken breast. Do not cut all the way through, as you will be filling the slits.

3. Drizzle the olive oil on top of each chicken breast, and then rub with paprika and salt.

4. Add the cream cheese to a large bowl and microwave for 45 seconds (be sure to cover the dish). Remove from the microwave and stir in the cheddar cheese and diced jalapenos.

5. Stuff each slit in the chicken with the jalapeno-cheese mixture.

6. Bake for about 30 minutes, or until chicken is fully cooked.

Nutrition: 424 calories, 26g total fat, 42g protein, 3g carbohydrates, 0g fiber, 444mg sodium

Carb count: **0**

Chicken Caprese Spaghetti Squash Boats

Yield: 4 (½ squash) servings | Prep time: 8 minutes | Cook time: 40 minutes

2 spaghetti squashes

1 tablespoon olive oil

¼ teaspoon pink Himalayan salt

½ teaspoon black pepper

2 (10-ounce) chicken breasts, diced

1 dry pint cherry tomatoes

1 (8-ounce) package mini mozzarella balls

1 handful of chopped fresh basil, to garnish

store-bought or homemade balsamic glaze, to garnish

1. Preheat the oven to 425°F.

2. Microwave each spaghetti squash separately for about 3 minutes to soften them. Cut each spaghetti squash in half and scrape out the seeds. Drizzle with olive oil, salt, and pepper. Bake for 15 minutes. (If you prefer to microwave the spaghetti squash for a second time, see Garlic Parm Spaghetti Squash on page 116 for directions.)

3. Once you remove from the oven, scrape out the flesh with a fork. Do not remove the flesh; keep it in the spaghetti squash. At this point, the spaghetti squash is not cooked through fully.

4. Top the squash with chicken, and then bake for another 10 minutes. Remove from oven. Add cherry tomatoes and mozzarella cheese. Bake for another 10 to 12 minutes until cheese is melted.

5. Garnish with chopped basil and balsamic glaze.

Nutrition: 250 calories, 13g total fat, 29g protein, 5g carbohydrates, 1g fiber, 241mg sodium

Carb count: **0**

Italian Sausage and Seasoned Veggies

Yield: 6 servings | Prep time: 12 minutes | Cook time: 30 minutes

2 cups halved baby carrots

2 red potatoes, diced

1 medium zucchini, halved then sliced into half coins

2 red peppers, cut into medium-size chunks

1 head broccoli, cut into florets

16 ounces Italian chicken sausage, sliced into coins

½ tablespoon dried basil

½ tablespoon dried oregano

½ tablespoon dried parsley

½ tablespoon garlic powder

½ tablespoon onion powder

½ tablespoon dried thyme

⅛ teaspoon red pepper flakes

5 tablespoons avocado oil

⅓ cup grated Parmesan cheese

handful fresh chopped basil, to top

1. Preheat the oven to 400°F.

2. Line a baking sheet with parchment paper. Add veggies and sausage in an even layer.

3. In a small bowl, combine all of the seasonings with the avocado oil. Pour the mixture onto the baking sheet and toss ingredients to coat.

4. Bake for about 15 minutes. Stir and bake for another 15 minutes, or until cooked to desired crispiness.

5. Remove from oven and top with grated Parmesan cheese and basil.

Nutrition: 375 calories, 21g total fat, 25g protein, 23g carbohydrates, 5g fiber, 443mg sodium

Carb count: **1½**

Cauliflower Grits & Shrimp

Yield: 4 servings | Prep time: 10 minutes | Cook time: 18 minutes

4 slices cooked turkey bacon, chopped

1 cauliflower head

1 pound shrimp, peeled and deveined

2½ tablespoons avocado oil

1 tablespoon Cajun spice

½ cup diced onion

2 garlic cloves, minced

1 cup grated cheddar cheese

¼ cup chopped scallions

1. Cut cauliflower into florets. Process in food processor to rice consistency. Measure out 4 cups and set aside.

2. To a bowl, add shrimp, 1½ tablespoons avocado oil, and Cajun spice. Stir to combine and set aside.

3. Heat remaining 1 tablespoon of avocado oil in a pan over medium-high heat. Add onion and garlic. Sauté for about 3 minutes. Add cauliflower rice to pan and stir to combine. Cover and cook for about 6 minutes.

4. Stir cheese into cauliflower rice. Melt for about 1 minute and then transfer to a serving dish.

5. Add shrimp to the skillet. Cook both sides until cooked through (until it turns pink), about 8 minutes total.

6. Spoon shrimp over cauliflower rice. Top with bacon bits and chopped scallions.

Nutrition: 359 calories, 21g total fat, 35g protein, 9g carbohydrates, 3g fiber, 590mg sodium

Carb count: ½

Garlic Parm Spaghetti Squash

Yield: 2 (½-squash) servings | Prep time: 7 minutes | Cook time: 20 minutes

1 spaghetti squash, halved lengthwise, seeds scraped out with a spoon

1 tablespoon avocado oil

1 tablespoon butter

3 cloves garlic, minced

1 cup low-sodium chicken stock

½ cup grated Parmesan cheese

⅓ cup sour cream

½ teaspoon black pepper

2 tablespoons finely chopped basil

1. Place spaghetti squash halves in a microwave-safe dish with the skin facing up. Add 1 inch of water and microwave for 12 to 15 minutes, until the squash is tender. Separate the strings with a fork and transfer to a bowl. Set aside. (If you prefer to bake spaghetti squash in oven, see Chicken Caprese Spaghetti Squash Boats on page 113 for directions.)

2. While the spaghetti squash is cooking, heat the avocado oil and butter in a pan over medium heat. Add the minced garlic; stir for 1 minute. Add the chicken stock. Increase heat to high, and bring stock to a boil then reduce heat to simmer and add the spaghetti squash. Cook for 2 to 3 minutes over medium heat.

3. Then, turn off the heat and add the Parmesan cheese. Stir until completely melted, about 1 minute. Add the sour cream, and stir again.

4. Transfer spaghetti squash to a serving dish. Garnish with pepper and basil.

Nutrition: 294 calories, 27g total fat, 11g protein, 5g carbohydrates, 1g fiber, 100mg sodium

Carb count: **0**

Crispy Chicken Parm

Yield: 4 servings | Prep time: 8 minutes | Cook time: 12 minutes

8 tablespoons butter, divided

½ cup Italian breadcrumbs (or homemade breadcrumbs made with crushed crackers)

½ cup plus 1 tablespoon grated Parmesan cheese, divided

¼ cup garbanzo bean flour

4 (5-ounce) chicken breasts, pounded thin

2 medium zucchini, sliced into coins

1. Melt 4 tablespoons of butter in a medium bowl.

2. In another bowl, combine breadcrumbs, Parmesan cheese, and flour. Dip the chicken in the butter first and then in the breadcrumb mixture. Repeat with all 4 chicken breasts, and set aside.

3. In a large skillet, heat 2 tablespoons butter over medium heat and then add the chicken. Cook each side for about 4 minutes, until the outside is crispy and the chicken is cooked through. Set aside.

4. Add the remaining 2 tablespoons of butter to the skillet. Add the zucchini and sauté until tender, about 4 minutes. Top zucchini with 1 tablespoon of Parmesan cheese. Transfer to a serving dish and serve immediately with chicken.

Nutrition: 498 calories, 29g total fat, 37g protein, 16g carbohydrates, 3g fiber, 559mg sodium

Carb count: **1**

Spinach Stuffed Pork Chops

Yield: 4 servings | Prep time: 7 minutes | Cook time: 40 minutes

1 (24-ounce) package boneless, center-cut pork chops (package should contain 4 chops)

1 (8-ounce) package cream cheese

½ cup grated Parmesan cheese

1 cup chopped spinach

3 cloves garlic, minced

1 tablespoon parsley, dried

1 tablespoon basil, dried

1. Preheat the oven to 350°F.

2. Slice a 3-inch pocket into each pork chop.

3. In a small bowl, mix the cream cheese, Parmesan cheese, spinach, garlic, parsley, and basil.

4. Stuff each pork chop with the mixture. Seal the edges with a fork.

5. Bake the pork chops for about 40 minutes.

Nutrition: 447 calories, 29g total fat, 43g protein, 5g carbohydrates, 0g fiber, 600mg sodium

Carb count: **0**

Sesame Shrimp with Brown Rice

Yield: 4 servings | Prep time: 6 minutes | Cook time: 13 minutes plus 30 minutes to marinate

1 pound large shrimp, peeled and deveined

¼ cup low-sodium soy sauce

3 garlic cloves, minced

2 limes, juiced

2 tablespoons rice wine vinegar

2 tablespoons avocado oil, divided

zero-carb sweetener, optional

2 cups cooked brown rice

2 avocados, halved, sliced

chopped green scallions and sesame seeds, for garnish, optional

1. In a large bowl, mix shrimp, soy sauce, garlic, lime juice, rice wine vinegar, 1 tablespoon avocado oil, and zero-carb sweetener, if using. Stir until shrimp is coated well. Cover bowl and set in fridge for 30 minutes.

2. Once shrimp is done marinating, heat avocado oil over medium-high heat in a skillet. Remove pieces of shrimp from bowl and heat in skillet for about 6 minutes, or until pink. Remove the shrimp and set aside.

3. Add the marinade from the mixing bowl to the same skillet. Simmer until sauce thickens to syrup consistency, about 4 minutes. Add the shrimp back to the skillet; toss and brown for about 3 minutes. Remove shrimp from heat.

4. Add ½ cup cooked brown rice to each of 4 plates. Add half an avocado, sliced, to each plate.

5. Evenly distribute shrimp over brown rice. Garnish with optional scallions and sesame seeds. Serve immediately.

Nutrition: 362 calories, 18g total fat, 33g protein, 31g carbohydrates, 6g fiber, 650mg sodium

Carb count: **2**

Cheesy Chicken Foil Packet

Yield: 4 servings | Prep time: 5 minutes | Cook time: 35 minutes plus 1 hour to refrigerate

2 tablespoons avocado oil

1 tablespoon balsamic vinegar

½ teaspoon pink Himalayan salt

½ teaspoon black pepper

4 (5-ounce) boneless, skinless chicken breasts

2 slices bacon, crumbled

8 tablespoons Annie's barbecue sauce

1 cup shredded cheddar cheese

½ cup diced tomatoes

¼ cup diced scallions

2 avocados, halved, sliced

1. In a large zip-top bag, combine the oil, vinegar, salt, and pepper. Add the chicken to the bag and seal. Massage to evenly coat the chicken. Refrigerate for at least 1 hour.

2. Preheat the oven to 400°F.

3. Cook bacon according to package directions.

4. Once the chicken is done marinating, grease a large piece of tin foil. Add 1 chicken breast and top with 2 tablespoons barbecue sauce. Wrap the foil around the chicken so it is completely enclosed. Repeat with the remaining chicken.

5. Bake for 30 minutes or until cooked through.

6. Open the foil packs and top each with ¼ cup shredded cheese and ¼ of the crumbled bacon. Put back in oven for 5 minutes (leaving the foil open), until cheese has melted.

7. Remove from oven and top each chicken breast evenly with diced tomatoes, scallions, and avocado.

Nutrition: 587 calories, 36g total fat, 43g protein, 25g carbohydrates, 6g fiber, 610mg sodium

Carb count: **1½**

Chicken Fajita Foil Packets

Yield: 2 (2-packet) servings | Prep time: 8 minutes | Cook time: 20 minutes

1 pound boneless, skinless chicken breasts, cut into thin fajita-style strips

2 bell peppers, sliced into thin strips

1 medium onion, sliced into thin strips

2 tablespoons avocado oil

1 packet taco seasoning

handful cilantro, chopped

4 Ezekiel brand corn tortillas

Toppings (optional):

guacamole

salsa

sour cream

lime wedges

hot sauce

1. Preheat the oven to 425°F.

2. In a large bowl, combine chicken, bell peppers, onion, avocado oil, taco seasoning, and cilantro.

3. Grease four 12-inch pieces of tin foil. Evenly divide the chicken mixture to the foil pieces. Wrap the foil around the chicken pieces so they are completely enclosed. Place foil packets on baking tray and cook for about 20 minutes or until chicken is cooked through.

4. Serve on 2 dishes, with 2 foil packets and 2 corn tortillas on each dish. Add desired toppings and serve immediately.

Nutrition: 496 calories, 22g total fat, 48g protein, 34g carbohydrates, 7g fiber, 579mg sodium

Carb count: **2**

Note: Use only 1 tortilla to lower carb count.

Peanut Zoodles

Yield: 4 servings | Prep time: 15 minutes | Cook time: 10 minutes

For the zoodles:

2 tablespoons sesame oil

2 teaspoons chopped garlic

1 cup shredded carrots

1 cup thinly sliced cabbage

1 red bell pepper, thinly sliced

3 large zucchini, spiralized into zoodles

For the peanut sauce:

½ cup creamy peanut butter

¼ cup honey

⅓ cup low-sodium soy sauce

2 tablespoons sesame oil

2 tablespoons rice vinegar

2 teaspoons minced fresh ginger

2 teaspoons hot sauce

Toppings:

1 tablespoon sesame seeds

handful cilantro, chopped

½ cup crushed peanuts

2 scallions, chopped

1. Heat the sesame oil and garlic in a large skillet over medium heat. Add the carrots, cabbage, and pepper slices; sauté for about 5 minutes or until veggies are tender. Add the zoodles and cook for about 3 minutes, until the zucchini is slightly softer. Turn off heat and set aside.

2. Combine the peanut sauce ingredients in a small saucepan over low heat. Whisk until the peanut butter is melted and the ingredients are well-combined, about 2 minutes.

3. Once the sauce is finished, pour it over the zoodles. Toss to combine.

4. Serve topped with sesame seeds, cilantro, peanuts, and scallions.

Nutrition: 459 calories, 31g total fat, 12g protein, 31g carbohydrates, 5g fiber, 690mg sodium

Carb count: **2**

Cashew Chicken with Veggies

Yield: 4 servings | Prep time: 10 minutes | Cook time: 20 minutes

1 tablespoon sesame oil

1 pound boneless, skinless chicken breast, diced into 1-inch cubes

1 carrot, chopped

1 tablespoon minced ginger

2 cloves garlic, minced

2 tablespoons low-sodium soy sauce

1 tablespoon sriracha

1 tablespoon honey

1 red bell pepper, diced

1 yellow onion, diced

1 head broccoli, cut into florets

½ cup crushed cashews

sesame seeds and chopped scallions, to garnish, optional

1. Heat sesame oil in a skillet over medium-high heat. Add chicken; sauté for 7 minutes or until browned. Add carrot, ginger, garlic, soy sauce, sriracha, and honey. Cook for another 5 minutes, until carrots soften. Add in red pepper, onion, and broccoli. Place lid on top of skillet; steam for another 7 minutes.

2. Stir in cashews; combine well. Remove from heat and divide mixture between 4 bowls. Garnish with optional sesame seeds and scallions.

Nutrition: 290 calories, 14g total fat, 27g protein, 15g carbohydrates, 2g fiber, 628mg sodium

Carb count: **1**

Ranch Quinoa Kale Bowl

Yield: 4 servings | Prep time: 25 minutes | Cook time: 0 minutes

For the ranch dressing:

1 cup sour cream

¼ cup organic milk

2 teaspoons lemon juice

2 teaspoons fresh or dried parsley

1 clove garlic, minced

1 tablespoon dried onion

¼ teaspoon pink Himalayan salt

½ teaspoon black pepper

For the kale bowl:

2 cups cooked quinoa

2 cups finely chopped kale

1 cup halved cherry tomatoes

1 cup cucumbers, chopped

2 avocados, halved, sliced

1. Blend all ranch dressing ingredients in a blender or food processor.

2. Mix the quinoa and kale and divide evenly between four serving bowls. Evenly divide the cherry tomatoes, cucumbers, and avocado between the four bowls. Drizzle with ranch dressing (you will likely have leftover dressing).

Nutrition: 400 calories, 23g total fat, 7g protein, 36g carbohydrates, 10g fiber, 360mg sodium

Carb count: **2**

Turkey, Bacon, & Swiss Lettuce Wrap

Yield: 4 servings | Prep time: 6 minutes | Cook time: 5 minutes

¼ pound sliced turkey breast

4 large romaine lettuce leaves

4 teaspoons avocado oil mayonnaise

8 slices bacon, cooked

8 slices Swiss cheese

1 tomato, thinly sliced into 8 slices

2 cups fresh strawberries

olive oil and vinegar or dressing of your choice, optional

1. Heat turkey in pan or oven to desired heat to decrease risk of listeria contamination.

2. Lay out romaine leaves. Spread 1 teaspoon of mayo onto each leaf. Top each leaf with 2 slices of heated turkey breast, 2 slices of bacon, 2 slices of cheese, and 2 tomato slices. Add dressing to wraps, if desired.

3. Roll the 4 lettuce wraps into a burrito shape and place on a dish. Add a side of ½ cup strawberries to each dish.

Nutrition: 310 calories, 22g total fat, 20g protein, 7g carbohydrates, 2g fiber, 538mg sodium

Carb count: ½

Wedge Salad

Yield: 2 servings | Prep time: 15 minutes | Cook time: 0 minutes

For the dressing:

¼ cup plain Greek yogurt

3 tablespoons sour cream

1 tablespoon mayonnaise

3 tablespoons organic milk

dash Worcestershire sauce

¼ cup pasteurized cheese crumbles (cheese of your choice)

2 teaspoons white balsamic vinegar

For the salad:

2 wedges iceberg lettuce

4 strips bacon, cooked and crumbled

4 hard-boiled eggs, chopped into pieces

10 grape tomatoes, sliced in half

1. In a small bowl, whisk dressing ingredients together. Set aside.

2. Place each iceberg lettuce wedge on a separate plate. Drizzle with the dressing. Evenly divide the bacon, eggs, and tomatoes between each wedge.

Nutrition: 350 calories, 22g total fat, 20g protein, 10g carbohydrates, 2g fiber, 451mg sodium

Carb count: ½

Chicken Spring Roll Bowl

Yield: 4 servings | Prep time: 10 minutes | Cook time: 12 minutes

¼ cup coconut oil

2 (6-ounce) boneless, skinless chicken breasts

4 hard-boiled eggs, chopped

1 cup chopped peanuts

4 radishes, shredded

4 teaspoons garlic powder

2 teaspoons black pepper

2 teaspoons fresh minced ginger

2 teaspoons dry mustard

4 cups shredded cabbage/coleslaw/carrot mixture (can be found premade in the supermarket)

1. In a skillet, heat coconut oil over medium heat. Add chicken and pan-fry both sides until cooked through, about 12 minutes. Once done, turn heat off and take chicken out of the pan to shred.

2. To a medium bowl, add the chicken, eggs, peanuts, radishes, all seasonings, and cabbage/carrot mixture. Stir until well-combined, then remove from heat.

Nutrition: 340 calories, 23g total fat, 27g protein, 7g carbohydrates, 2g fiber, 118mg sodium

Carb count: ½

Mozzarella Chicken & Spinach Skillet

Yield: 4 servings | Prep time: 5 minutes | Cook time: 9 minutes

- 3 tablespoons butter
- 8 cups frozen spinach, thawed
- 2 cans organic canned chicken
- 1 pint cherry tomatoes, halved
- 4 teaspoons black pepper
- 4 teaspoons fresh chopped basil
- 2 cups shredded mozzarella cheese

1. Melt butter in a skillet over medium-low heat. Add spinach evenly and cook until heated well, about 2 minutes.

2. Once the spinach is done, add chicken, tomatoes, pepper, and basil.

3. Cook for about 6 minutes, or to desired temperature, then add cheese and melt for 1 minute.

Nutrition: 370 calories, 23g total fat, 31g protein, 8g carbohydrates, 3g fiber, 472mg sodium

Carb count: ½

Chicken Broccoli Alfredo

Yield: 4 servings | Prep time: 5 minutes | Cook time: 12 minutes

1 pound chicken breast, diced into ½-inch-thick cubes

½ teaspoon black pepper

1 teaspoon parsley, dried

2 teaspoons garlic powder

¼ cup butter plus additional for greasing the pan

8 ounces cream cheese

2 cups heavy cream

2 cups shredded Parmesan cheese

4 cups cooked broccoli

1. Place diced chicken in a bowl and season with pepper, parsley, and garlic.

2. Melt the greasing butter in pan over medium heat. Add chicken to the pan; cook until the outsides are browned and the inside is no longer pink, about 10 minutes.

3. To make the alfredo sauce, melt ¼ cup of butter over medium heat in a saucepan. Add the cream cheese; combine with whisk until smooth. Add heavy cream and stir all ingredients together for 30 seconds. Then, stir in the Parmesan cheese for an additional 1 minute. Remove pan from heat.

4. Add the cooked chicken into the sauce.

5. Serve over steamed broccoli.

Nutrition: 685 calories, 38g total fat, 29g protein, 11g carbohydrates, 2g fiber, 595mg sodium

Carb count: **1**

Lettuce-Wrapped Fish Tacos

Yield: 4 servings | Prep time: 8 minutes | Cook time: 25 minutes

4 (5-ounce) fresh cod fillets

2 tablespoons avocado oil

2 cups coleslaw mix

¾ cup avocado oil mayonnaise

3 tablespoons lime juice

1 teaspoon fresh chopped basil

1 teaspoon fresh chopped cilantro

1 teaspoon black pepper

¼ teaspoon pink Himalayan salt

4 romaine lettuce leaves

3 radishes, thinly sliced

1 avocado, cubed

1. Preheat the oven to 425°F. Place cod fillets on baking sheet and drizzle with avocado oil.

2. Bake fish for about 25 minutes, or until they flake with a fork.

3. To make a homemade aioli, in a small bowl, combine mayonnaise, lime juice, basil, cilantro, pepper, and salt. Set aside.

4. Once fish is done, place each fillet on lettuce leaf. Top each with the aioli, radishes, and diced avocado.

Nutrition: 550 calories, 35g total fat, 27g protein, 6g carbohydrates, 4g fiber, 542mg sodium

Carb count: **½**

Stuffed Sprouted-Grain Quesadillas

Yield: 4 (½-quesadilla) servings | Prep time: 5 minutes | Cook time: 10 minutes

1 green bell pepper, diced

1 yellow onion, diced

2 tablespoons avocado oil, divided

2 cups cooked chicken (premade, canned, or rotisserie)

2 teaspoons chopped jalapeno

4 Ezekiel sprouted grain tortillas

2 tablespoons Primal Kitchen ranch dressing

4 tablespoons diced tomatoes, diced

1 cup shredded cheddar cheese

1. In a skillet over medium heat, sauté green peppers and onion with 1 tablespoon of the avocado oil until the onions are translucent, about 2 minutes. Add the chicken and jalapeno and heat for 3 minutes. Then, remove from pan and set aside.

2. Add the second tablespoon of avocado oil to a separate pan to coat, and heat over medium heat. Lay 1 tortilla in the pan, and add ½ of the chicken and veggie mixture, ranch dressing, tomatoes, and cheese. Lay the second tortilla on top. Let the tortilla brown and then flip to brown the other side. Repeat with the remaining ingredients to make a second quesadilla.

3. Cut each quesadilla in half to serve.

Nutrition: 476 calories, 25g total fat, 36g protein, 25g carbohydrates, 7g fiber, 423mg sodium

Carb count: **1½**

Sesame Beef & Broccoli

Yield: 4 servings | Prep time: 5 minutes | Cook time: 22 minutes

4 tablespoons coconut oil

1½ pounds sirloin steak, sliced into strips

4 garlic cloves, minced

1 tablespoon freshly grated ginger

4 cups broccoli florets

2 tablespoons Bragg's liquid coconut aminos

2 tablespoons sesame seed oil

2 tablespoons honey

sesame seeds, to garnish

1. Heat the coconut oil in a large pan over medium-high heat. Add the sirloin, and sear each side for about 7 minutes.

2. Reduce the heat to medium-low and add the garlic, ginger, and broccoli. Sauté for about 5 minutes, then add in the coconut aminos, sesame oil, and honey. Heat for about 3 minutes.

3. Remove beef and broccoli from heat. Place in serving dish and top with sesame seeds.

Nutrition: 514 calories, 34g total fat, 39g protein, 15g carbohydrates, 2g fiber, 598mg sodium

Carb count: **1**

Egg Salad Sandwiches

Yield: 4 servings | Prep time: 5 minutes | Cook time: 8 to 10 minutes

8 eggs

¼ cup avocado oil mayonnaise

1 teaspoon Dijon mustard

½ teaspoon yellow mustard

2 teaspoons lemon juice

¼ cup chopped scallions

½ teaspoon black pepper

4 pieces Ezekiel sprouted flax bread

1. Gently place the eggs in a saucepan. Cover with cold water. Bring water to a boil, about 8 to 10 minutes, then remove from heat. Cover the saucepan and let the eggs stand in hot water for about 10 minutes.

2. Remove the eggs from the hot water and run cold water over them. Allow them to cool (or place in ice bath to speed up cooling process), and then peel. Chop the eggs into chunks and place in medium bowl.

3. In a separate small bowl, mix together the mayonnaise, both mustards, lemon juice, and chopped scallions. Scoop the mixture into the bowl with the eggs. Add pepper and stir all ingredients to combine.

4. Toast 4 pieces of Ezekiel bread, then evenly divide egg salad mixture.

Nutrition: 384 calories, 23g total fat, 19g protein, 28g carbohydrates, 7g fiber, 374mg sodium

Carb count: **1½**

Salmon Avocado Cucumber Bites

Yield: 2 servings | Prep time: 6 minutes | Cook time: 0 minutes

1 (5-ounce) can salmon

1 avocado, pitted and halved

2 handfuls fresh dill, chopped

1 medium cucumber, cut into medium-sized coins

½ cup walnuts, divided

1. Drain canned salmon; set aside.

2. In a medium bowl, mash avocado halves with a fork. Add the canned salmon and dill. Mix until well-combined.

3. Top each cucumber coin with 1 tablespoon of the salmon avocado mixture until you run out.

4. Divide the salmon avocado cucumber bites between two plates, with a side of ¼ cup walnuts on each.

Nutrition: 430 calories, 29g total fat, 23g protein, 12g carbohydrates, 7g fiber, 307mg sodium

Carb count: ½

Almond-Crusted Pork Chops

Yield: 4 servings | Prep time: 5 minutes | Cook time: 15 minutes

4 cups baby carrots

2 large eggs

1⅓ cups almond meal

2 tablespoons Mrs. Dash garlic herb seasoning, or seasoning mixture of your choice

4 tablespoons coconut oil

4 (5-ounce) pork chops

1. Place baby carrots in a covered microwave-safe dish. Add 1/2 cup of water. Microwave for 6 minutes, or to your desired tenderness. Let stand, covered, for 5 minutes longer.

2. In a large bowl, add both eggs and beat with a fork.

3. In a separate bowl, add the almond meal and seasoning; combine.

4. In a large pan, heat coconut oil over medium-high heat.

5. Take one pork chop and dip it into the egg mixture; coat both sides. Then dip the pork chop into almond meal and seasoning mixture; coat both sides well. If only one pork chop can fit in your pan, gently place it in the hot pan and begin cooking. If multiple pork chops can fit in your pan, season and coat them and place them in the pan at once.

6. Cook each side until nicely browned and the internal temperature reaches 145°F, about 15 minutes per pork chop. Repeat process with remaining pork chops.

7. Plate each pork chop on a dish with a side of 1 cup of cooked carrots.

Nutrition: 384 calories, 23g total fat, 29g protein, 12g carbohydrates, 4g fiber, 178mg sodium

Carb count: **1**

Cabbage & Onion Egg Scramble

Yield: 4 servings | Prep time: 3 minutes | Cook time: 11 minutes

2 tablespoons coconut oil

½ cup chopped yellow onion

4 cups shredded cabbage

10 eggs, beaten

½ teaspoon black pepper

1 cup sauerkraut

2 avocados, pitted and halved

1. Heat coconut oil in a pan over medium heat. Add onion and sauté until browned, about 5 minutes. Add shredded cabbage and sauté until soft, about 3 minutes. Add beaten eggs and pepper; scramble until cooked, about 3 minutes.

2. Divide scramble between four plates. Top each plate with ¼ cup sauerkraut and ½ avocado.

Nutrition: 400 calories, 28g total fat, 20g protein, 14g carbohydrates, 9g fiber, 559mg sodium

Carb count: ½

Desserts

As I've mentioned earlier, there are always healthy swaps to your favorite not-so-healthy foods. Dessert equals sugar, right? Not always. These recipes contain clever ways to satisfy a sweet tooth without elevating your blood sugar levels. These GDM desserts do not contain foods with "sugar-free" ingredients, unlike most other GDM desert recipes. "Sugar-free" is typically a sign that artificial sweeteners are used such as sucralose, commonly known as Splenda. These recipes, however, contain real-food ingredients, such as fruit, or zero-carb sweeteners from plants, such as stevia. Sometimes all it takes to drastically change the nutrition content of a meal is changing a few ingredients, such as quinoa flour instead of white flour or Stevia instead of white sugar.

Peanut Butter Cookies

Yield: 9 (2-cookie) servings | Prep time: 5 minutes, plus 10 minutes to freeze

⅔ cup natural peanut butter

2 tablespoons softened butter

1 cup unsweetened natural shredded coconut

4 drops vanilla-flavored stevia

1. In a medium bowl, add peanut butter to softened butter. Stir. Add coconut and stevia; mix well.

2. Spoon onto a sheet pan lined with parchment paper. Freeze for 10 minutes.

3. Serve, or keep stored in refrigerator, tightly bagged.

Nutrition: 200 calories, 16 g total fat, 6g protein, 10 g carbohydrates, 3g fiber, 86mg sodium

Carb count: ½

Peanut Butter Fluff

Yield: 8 servings | Prep time: 7 minutes, plus at least 6 hours to refrigerate

½ cup heavy whipping cream

4 ounces softened cream cheese

2¼ tablespoons natural peanut butter

5 tablespoons Swerve Confectioners sweetener

½ teaspoon vanilla extract

1 teaspoon raw cacao nibs or unsweetened chocolate chips

1. In a medium bowl, beat the heavy whipping cream for about 2 minutes with a mixer until it turns to whipped cream.

2. In a separate bowl, use a mixer to beat the softened cream cheese, peanut butter, Swerve Confectioners sweetener, and vanilla. Beat for about 2 minutes or until smooth and creamy, then add the whipped cream. Mix on low for 30 seconds until combined and smooth.

3. Top mixture with cacao nibs or unsweetened chocolate chips.

4. Refrigerate for at least 6 hours, then serve.

Nutrition: 125 calories, 13g total fat, 2g protein, 9g carbohydrates, 0g fiber, 78mg sodium

Carb count: ½

Although the Nutrition Facts label of Swerve Confectioners sweetener reads 3 grams of carbohydrates, erythritol does not impact blood sugar levels, so carb count is technically lower than ½.

Chocolate Mousse

Yield: 6 servings | Prep time: 5 minutes, plus 30 minutes to refrigerate

4 tablespoons softened butter

2 ounces softened cream cheese

1 tablespoon raw cacao powder or cocoa powder

3 ounces heavy whipping cream

1. Add the softened butter and cream cheese to a medium bowl. Mix with a whisk until smooth.

2. Add cacao powder and mix again.

3. In a separate bowl, whip the heavy cream with a mixer. Then slowly add to the cream cheese mixture.

4. Spoon into 4 small bowls. Refrigerate for at least 30 minutes before serving.

Nutrition: 153 calories, 17g total fat, 1g protein, 1g carbohydrates, 0g fiber, 117mg sodium

Carb count: **0**

3-Ingredient No-Bake Coconut Cookies

Yield: 20 cookies | Prep time: 7 minutes, plus 1 hour to refrigerate

3 cups shredded unsweetened coconut flakes

1 cup melted coconut oil

½ cup monk fruit–sweetened maple syrup

1. Line a large plate with parchment paper.

2. In a medium mixing bowl, combine all the ingredients. Mix well.

3. Lightly wet your hands (to prevent sticking). Form small balls with the batter and place them 1 to 2 inches apart on the lined plate.

4. Press down onto each cookie with a fork. Refrigerate for 1 hour until firm.

Nutrition: 142 calories, 15g total fat, 1g protein, 2g carbohydrates, 2g fiber, 15mg sodium

Carb count: **0**

Chocolate Chip Quinoa Cookies

Yield: 12 cookies | Prep time: 8 minutes | Cook time: 10 minutes

1 cup quinoa flour

½ teaspoon baking powder

⅛ teaspoon pink Himalayan salt

1 teaspoon ground cinnamon

2 tablespoons coconut sugar

2 eggs

5 tablespoons melted coconut oil

2 teaspoons vanilla extract

⅓ cup unsweetened chocolate chips or raw cacao nibs

1. Preheat the oven to 350°F.

2. In a medium bowl, mix the quinoa flour, baking powder, salt, cinnamon, and sugar.

3. In a separate bowl, mix the eggs, oil, and vanilla.

4. Combine the wet ingredients with the dry ingredients. Add the chocolate chips. Mix until well-combined.

5. Dollop the batter onto a baking sheet lined with parchment paper to make 12 cookies.

6. Bake for about 10 minutes, or until your desired crispiness is reached.

7. Let cool on baking sheet for a few minutes.

Nutrition: 132 calories, 8g total fat, 3g protein, 13g carbohydrates, 3g fiber, 227mg sodium

Carb count: **1**

Blueberry Scones

Yield: 8 scones | Prep time: 8 minutes | Cook time: 12 to 18 minutes

½ cup coconut flour

½ cup almond flour

⅛ teaspoon pink Himalayan salt

¼ cup Truvia sweetener

2 teaspoons baking powder

1 cup fresh blueberries

½ cup unsalted, softened butter

½ cup heavy cream

2 eggs

2 teaspoons vanilla extract

1. Preheat the oven to 350°F.

2. In a large bowl, combine the coconut and almond flours, salt, Truvia, and baking powder. After mixing, stir in the blueberries.

3. Add the butter, heavy cream, eggs, and vanilla. Mix until well-combined.

4. With your hands, shape 2 tablespoons of dough into a triangular scone shape. You should make about 8 scones.

5. Place on a cookie sheet lined with parchment paper. Bake for 12 to 18 minutes or until the edges are golden.

6. Let cool then serve, or store in an airtight container.

Nutrition: 222 calories, 20g total fat, 3g protein, 15g carbohydrates, 10g fiber, 80mg sodium

Carb count: ½

5-Minute Strawberry Frozen Yogurt

Yield: 4 servings | Prep time: 5 minutes | Cook time: 0 minutes

4 cups frozen strawberries

2 tablespoons agave nectar

½ cup plain Greek yogurt

1 tablespoon fresh lemon juice

2 tablespoons chia seeds, divided

1. Add the frozen strawberries, agave nectar, yogurt, and lemon juice to a food processor. Process until creamy, about 4 to 5 minutes.

2. Serve immediately. Top each dish with ½ tablespoon of chia seeds.

Nutrition: 79 calories, 2g total fat, 4g protein, 13g carbohydrates, 3g fiber, 13mg sodium

Carb count: **1**

Snickerdoodle Cookie Balls

Yield: 5 (2-ball) servings | Prep time: 7 minutes, plus 1 to 2 hours to refrigerate

½ cup almond butter

2½ teaspoons ground cinnamon, divided

3 tablespoons coconut flour

3 tablespoons coconut milk

6 tablespoons xylitol, divided

15 drops vanilla liquid stevia

½ teaspoon organic vanilla extract

⅛ teaspoon pink Himalayan salt

1. Place almond butter, 1 teaspoon cinnamon, coconut flour, coconut milk, 3 tablespoons xylitol, liquid stevia, vanilla extract, and salt into a bowl. Mix until well-combined.

2. Roll into balls.

3. Mix 1½ teaspoons cinnamon and 3 tablespoons xylitol and in a small bowl. Roll cookie balls in the cinnamon mixture to coat.

4. Refrigerate for 1 to 2 hours, and then enjoy. Cookie balls can be stored in the refrigerator.

Nutrition: 201 calories, 15g total fat, 5g protein, 15g carbohydrates, 3g fiber, 54mg sodium

Carb count: **1**

Chocolate Chip Skillet Cookie

Yield: 12 servings | Prep time: 5 minutes | Cook time: 27 to 32 minutes

½ cup butter

1 large egg

1 teaspoon vanilla extract

2 tablespoons coconut sugar

¼ cup Swerve Granular sweetener

2 cups almond flour

¼ teaspoon pink Himalayan salt

½ cup sugar-free Lily's Dark Chocolate Premium chocolate chips, divided

1. Preheat the oven to 350°F.

2. Heat the butter in a 9-inch cast-iron skillet over high heat until bubbling. Reduce heat to low, cover pan, and continue to cook butter until it begins to brown, about 2 minutes. Once browned, remove from heat and let cool for 5 minutes.

3. While butter is cooling, whisk the egg and vanilla in a medium bowl. Add the coconut sugar and Swerve Granular sweetener. Mix well. Add the butter, and mix again.

4. Slowly add in the almond flour, salt, and half of the chocolate chips. Mix until well-combined (the consistency should be slightly thicker than cookie dough).

5. Spoon the batter into skillet. Top with the remaining chocolate chips.

6. Bake for 25 to 30 minutes or until a toothpick inserted in the center comes out clean.

7. Cut into 12 slices, and serve.

Nutrition: 141 calories, 14g total fat, 2g protein, 14g carbohydrates, 3g fiber, 426mg sodium

Carb count: **1***

* Carbohydrate effect on blood sugar may be lower; erythritol is an ingredient in Lily's chocolate chip cookies that is counted toward grams of carbohydrates but does not impact blood sugar levels.

No-Bake Coconut Delights

Yield: 10 servings | Prep time: 7 minutes, plus 30 minutes to firm

3 cups unsweetened shredded coconut

⅓ cup coconut oil

½ cup Granular Swerve sweetener

2 teaspoons vanilla extract

⅓ teaspoon pink Himalayan salt

2 tablespoons unsweetened chocolate chips

2 tablespoons finely chopped walnuts

1. Place shredded coconut, coconut oil, Granular Swerve, vanilla extract, and salt in a food processor. Combine until the mixture is blended and sticky.

2. Form the mixture into desired shapes.

3. Sprinkle unsweetened chocolate chips and crushed nuts onto cookies.

4. Leave cookies at room temperature to firm up, at least 30 minutes. Cookies can be stored in fridge.

Nutrition: 207 calories, 21g total fat, 2g protein, 7g carbohydrates, 3g fiber, 62mg sodium

Carb count: ½

Gooey Skillet Brownie

Yield: 2 (½-skillet) servings | Prep time: 6 minutes | Cook time: 13 to 16 minutes

5 tablespoons almond flour

3 tablespoons cocoa powder

3 tablespoons Granular Swerve sweetener

1 teaspoon baking powder

3 tablespoons water

2 tablespoons melted butter

1 large egg

¼ teaspoon vanilla extract

1 tablespoon sugar-free chocolate chips

1. Preheat the oven to 325°F. Lightly grease a 6-inch skillet (or casserole dish).

2. In a medium bowl, whisk together almond flour, cocoa powder, sweetener, and baking powder.

3. Stir in the water, melted butter, egg, and vanilla extract until well-combined.

4. Pour the mixture into the skillet. Sprinkle with chocolate chips. Bake for 13 to 16 minutes, or until puffed. The brownie should jiggle slightly when shaken (or, cook longer, if preferred). Serve immediately.

Nutrition: 292 calories, 26g total fat, 9g protein, 11g carbohydrates, 5g fiber, 152 mg sodium

Carb count: ½

Snacks

Snacking is encouraged with GDM, as it will keep your blood sugar stable throughout the day. Snacking is also helpful for when you approach meal time, as you may not be ravenous and can focus on eating proper portions. Think of healthy snacks as mini-meals that provide your body with nutrients, compared to unhealthy snacks, which bring down your energy levels and can spike up your blood sugar. These snacks contain protein and healthy fats to keep you filled up and energized. Enjoy the variety of low-carb snacks offered in this chapter, from cheesy jalapeno mushroom bites to lime-roasted cashews.

Kale Chips

Yield: 3 servings | Prep time: 3 minutes | Cook time: 12 minutes

1 bunch kale, chopped

1 tablespoon lemon juice

2 tablespoons coconut oil

⅛ teaspoon pink Himalayan salt

1. Preheat the oven to 350°F.

2. Place all ingredients in a large bowl. Massage the lemon juice, oil, and salt into kale well.

3. Place on parchment-lined baking sheet and bake for about 12 minutes, or to desired crispiness. Be careful not to burn the kale chips.

Nutrition: 125 calories, 10g total fat, 4g protein, 8g carbohydrates, 3g fiber, 77 mg sodium

Carb count: ½

Avocado Crisps

Yield: 5 servings | Prep time: 3 minutes | Cook time: 15 to 17 minutes

1½ ripe avocados

⅛ teaspoon pink Himalayan salt

1¼ cups finely grated Parmesan cheese

1 lemon, zested

pinch black pepper

1. Preheat the oven to 350°F.

2. In a bowl, mix all of the ingredients together until well-combined.

3. Place teaspoon-sized dollops onto a baking tray lined with parchment paper. Flatten into thin disks.

4. Bake for 15 to 17 minutes, or until golden brown.

Nutrition: 192 calories, 15g total fat, 13g protein, 4g carbohydrates, 4g fiber, 555mg sodium

Carb count: **0**

Buffalo Chicken Celery Sticks

Yield: 6 (2-stick) servings | Prep time: 5 minutes | Cook time: 0 minutes

2 cups shredded chicken (use leftover chicken, rotisserie, or canned)

¼ cup avocado oil mayonnaise

½ teaspoon garlic powder

⅛ teaspoon pink Himalayan salt

¼ teaspoon black pepper

3 tablespoons buffalo sauce

6 celery stalks, halved (12 total)

chopped chives, to garnish

1. Mix the chicken, mayonnaise, garlic powder, salt, pepper, and buffalo sauce in a bowl.

2. Fill each celery stalk with the chicken mixture.

3. Garnish with chives.

Nutrition: 213 calories, 10g total fat, 25g protein, 3g carbohydrates, 2g fiber, 410 mg sodium

Carb count: **0**

Cheesy Jalapeno Mushroom Bites

Yield: 6 (2-piece) servings | Prep time: 8 minutes | Cook time: 20 minutes

8 ounces turkey bacon

12 cremini mushrooms, washed and de-stemmed, stems reserved

2 tablespoons butter

7 ounces cream cheese

4 tablespoons fresh jalapenos, finely chopped

½ cup shredded cheddar cheese

1 teaspoon paprika powder

1. Preheat the oven to 400°F.

2. Cook turkey bacon according to package directions. Let cool on plate, then shred to bite-sized pieces.

3. Place mushrooms on a greased baking dish.

4. Add the mushroom stems and butter to a sauté pan. Sauté until browned.

5. Once finished, add mushrooms stems to a small bowl and mix with the turkey bacon bits, cream cheese, jalapenos, shredded cheddar, and paprika. Spoon mixture into the mushrooms. Some excess mixture may spill over the mushrooms.

6. Bake for approximately 20 minutes, or until the stuffing has browned slightly.

Nutrition: 254 calories, 21g total fat, 14g protein, 4g carbohydrates, 0g fiber, 494mg sodium

Carb count: **0**

Parmesan Tomato Crisps

Yield: 6 servings | Prep time: 7 minutes | Cook time: 1 hour

6 cups beefsteak tomatoes, thinly sliced

2 tablespoons extra-virgin olive oil

1 teaspoons pink Himalayan salt

1 teaspoon garlic powder

2 tablespoons fresh chopped parsley

2 tablespoons grated Parmesan cheese

6 GG brand crispbread crackers

1. Preheat the oven to 200°F.

2. Toss the sliced tomatoes in the olive oil to coat. Place slices gently onto a baking pan.

3. In a small bowl, whisk together all the remaining ingredients except for the crackers. Sprinkle mixture over each tomato slice.

4. Leave in the oven for about 1 hour.

5. Add the tomato slices to the GG crispbread crackers. Serve immediately.

Nutrition: 119 calories, 5g total fat, 4g protein, 19g carbohydrates, 7g fiber, 459 mg sodium

Carb count: **1**

Note: You may have leftover tomato slices, depending on the amount you want on your cracker. If you will be eating additional GG crackers, it's important to calculate the additional amount of carbohydrates you will be consuming. These crackers have excellent fiber content, so be sure to subtract fiber from carbohydrates.

Hummus

Yield: 8 servings | Prep time: 5 minutes | Cook time: 0 minutes

2 cups canned low-sodium garbanzo beans, washed and drained

⅓ cup tahini

¼ cup lemon juice

1 teaspoon pink Himalayan salt

2 cloves garlic, minced

1 tablespoon olive oil

pinch paprika

raw veggies or GG brand crackers, to serve

Place all ingredients in food processor and process until desired consistency is reached. Serve with veggies and crackers, if desired.

Nutrition: 249 calories, 17g total fat, 9g protein, 15g carbohydrates, 5g fiber, 335mg sodium

Carb count: **1**

Tahini-Free Black Bean Hummus

Yield: 4 servings | Prep time: 5 minutes | Cook time: 0 minutes

1 (15-ounce) can low-sodium black beans, drained and rinsed

¼ cup fresh cilantro

3 garlic cloves, minced

½ teaspoon cumin

½ teaspoon paprika

1 tablespoon olive oil

1 lime, juiced

½ teaspoon pink Himalayan salt

raw veggies or GG brand crackers, to serve

Place all ingredients in food processor and process until desired consistency is reached. Serve with raw veggies or GG crackers, if desired.

Nutrition: 128 calories, 3g total fat, 6g protein, 18g carbohydrates, 5g fiber, 512mg sodium

Carb count: **1**

Lime-Roasted Cashews

Yield: 8 servings | Prep time: 2 minutes | Cook time: 20 to 25 minutes

2 cups salted cashews

1 tablespoon maple syrup

½ lime, juiced

1. Preheat the oven to 375°F.

2. Mix all ingredients in a bowl. Spread out on a baking sheet lined with parchment paper.

3. Bake for 20 to 25 minutes or to desired crispiness; stir occasionally.

Nutrition: 167 calories, 13g total fat, 5g protein, 10g carbohydrates, 1g fiber, 120mg sodium

Carb count: ½

Baked Cauliflower Tots

Yield: 4 servings | Prep time: 10 minutes | Cook time: 40 minutes

2 medium heads cauliflower, cut into florets

¼ cup diced onion

¼ cup grated Parmesan cheese

¼ cup finely ground breadcrumbs (can be store-bought or homemade from crushed crackers, such as Mary's Gone Crackers)

1 large egg

¼ teaspoon pink Himalayan salt

pinch black pepper

1. Preheat the oven to 350°F.

2. Line a baking sheet with parchment paper and grease the parchment paper.

3. Bring a large pot of water to a boil, and then add the cauliflower florets. Cook until fork-tender, about 7 minutes.

4. Drain the florets and transfer them to a food processor. Process for a few seconds until cauliflower is in rice-size pieces.

5. Add 3 cups of the cauliflower to a large bowl. Add onion, Parmesan cheese, breadcrumbs, egg, salt, and pepper. Mix until you've achieved a mashed-potato like consistency.

6. Mold 1 to 2 tablespoons of the mixture into desired shape (such as tater tots) until all the mixture is used up. Place each tot on a baking sheet about 1 inch apart.

7. Bake for 18 minutes and then flip and bake for an additional 15 minutes, or until crispy.

Nutrition: 126 calories, 4g total fat, 10g protein, 17g carbohydrates, 7g fiber, 226mg sodium

Carb count: **1**

Salt & Vinegar Zucchini Crisps

Yield: 2 servings | Prep time: 7 minutes | Cook time: 2 to 3 hours

4 cups (about 2 to 3 medium) thinly sliced zucchini

2 tablespoons avocado oil

2 tablespoons white balsamic vinegar

1 teaspoon pink Himalayan salt

1. Preheat the oven to 200°F.

2. Place zucchini in a large bowl.

3. In a separate small bowl, mix avocado oil, vinegar, and salt together. Add mixture to zucchini and toss.

4. Place the zucchini in even layers in a pan lined with parchment paper.

5. Depending on the thickness of the zucchini, cook time will be between 2 to 3 hours. Flip zucchini and rotate baking sheet halfway through.

Nutrition: 144 calories, 14g total fat, 0g protein, 5g carbohydrates, 0g fiber, 260mg sodium

Carb count: **0**

Cheesy Jalapeno Bites

Yield: 4 servings | Prep time: 5 minutes | Cook time: 20 minutes

1 cup feta cheese

½ teaspoon cumin

½ teaspoon chili powder

½ teaspoon paprika

½ teaspoon oregano, dried

¼ teaspoon pink Himalayan salt

10 jalapeno peppers, de-stemmed and de-seeded, halved lengthwise

1. Preheat the oven to 350°F. Line a baking sheet with parchment paper.

2. In a medium bowl, add all ingredients except for the jalapenos. Mix until well-combined.

3. Place each halved jalapeno on the baking sheet and fill with the cheese mixture.

4. Bake for about 20 minutes.

Nutrition: 112 calories, 8g total fat, 6g protein, 4g carbohydrates, 1g fiber, 385mg sodium

Carb count: **0**

Taco Cheese Crisps

Yield: 4 servings | Prep time: 5 minutes | Cook time: 25 to 30 minutes

6 slices Applegate cheddar cheese slices

2 to 3 teaspoons taco seasoning

1. Preheat the oven to 350°F.

2. Line a baking sheet with parchment paper.

3. Cut each cheese slice into 4 pieces to equal 24 squares. Place them about 1 inch apart on baking sheet.

4. Bake for 25 to 30 minutes, or to preferred crispiness. Sprinkle taco seasoning while crisps cool.

5. Allow crisps at least 5 minutes to cool, as they will continue to crisp.

Nutrition: 109 calories, 9g total fat, 8g protein, 1g carbohydrates, 0g fiber, 270mg sodium

Carb count: **0**

Warm Caprese Dip

Yield: 5 servings | Prep time: 3 minutes | Cook time: 17 minutes

10 ounces fresh mozzarella cheese

3 Roma tomatoes, seeded and juiced

3 tablespoons fresh chopped basil

GG brand crackers, for dipping

1. Preheat the oven to 375°F.

2. Chop up all ingredients and then add to a small baking dish. Bake for 15 minutes and then broil for 2 minutes on high to brown the cheese.

3. Serve with crackers, if desired.

Nutrition: 158 calories, 10g total fat, 11g protein, 4g carbohydrates, 1g fiber, 179mg sodium

Carb count: **0**

PB Celery Sticks

Yield: 1 serving | Prep time: 3 minutes | Cook time: 0 minutes

- 1 tablespoon natural peanut butter
- 2 (4-inch) celery sticks
- 1 tablespoon no-added-sugar dried cherries

Spread peanut butter onto celery sticks and sprinkle dried cherries on top.

Nutrition: 135 calories, 8g total fat, 4g protein, 10g carbohydrates, 1g fiber, 53mg sodium

Carb count: ½

Soft and Warm Pretzels

Yield: 12 servings | Prep time: 12 minutes | Cook time: 15 minutes

3 cups shredded mozzarella cheese

4 tablespoons cream cheese

2 teaspoons dried yeast

2 tablespoons warm water

1½ cups almond flour

2 teaspoons xanthan gum

2 eggs, room temperature

2 tablespoons melted butter, divided

1 tablespoon coarse salt

1. Preheat the oven to 400°F.

2. Line a baking sheet with parchment paper.

3. In a microwave-safe dish, microwave the mozzarella and cream cheese in 30-second increments (stirring in between) until fully melted.

4. Dissolve the yeast in the warm water. Let sit for 2 minutes to activate it.

5. With a mixer, mix almond flour and xanthan gum. Mix well. Add the eggs, yeast mixture, and 1 tablespoon of the melted butter. Mix again.

6. Add the hot melted cheese to the mixer. With the mixer, knead the dough until all ingredients are fully combined (about 5 minutes).

7. Split the dough into 12 balls. Roll each ball into a skinny log shape. Then, twist into pretzel shape. Place on the baking sheet. Brush the pretzels with the remaining butter and sprinkle the coarse salt.

8. Bake for about 12 minutes, or until golden brown.

Nutrition: 147 calories, 11g total fat, 10g protein, 2g carbohydrates, 1g fiber, 580mg sodium

Carb count: **0**

Appendix

Useful Kitchen Tools

Having useful kitchen tools on hand can make preparing meals far less daunting. Review the list of tools below and considering purchasing them or using the ones that have been stored in your cabinets to transform your cooking and reduce your prep time.

- Cast-iron skillet (if you have low iron levels, this is especially beneficial for you because safe amounts of iron will leach into your food)

- Dehydrator

- Food processor

- Glass baking dishes

- Immersion blender

- Mixer

- Natural ceramic skillet

- Salad spinner bowl

- Slow cooker and/or pressure cooker

- Quality knives

- Waffle maker

- Vitamix or high-speed blender

Meal Planning Chart

After trying the recipes in the book or developing your own with your newfound nutrition knowledge, keep a running list of your favorite meals and snacks. Include the grams of carbohydrates or carb count, or both, to ensure your meals are within your recommended daily carbohydrate limit. You may find it helpful to make a list on Sunday of the meals you'll be consuming for the week ahead, especially if you're meal prepping. Meal planning, preparation, and organization is key to succeeding in following a carbohydrate-controlled plan, or any diet plan for that matter.

Breakfast	Carbs (grams)	Carb count

Lunch	Carbs (grams)	Carb count

Dinner	Carbs (grams)	Carb count

Snacks	Carbs (grams)	Carb count

Grocery Shopping List

Non-Starchy Vegetables

- ❏ Alfalfa sprouts
- ❏ Artichokes
- ❏ Arugula
- ❏ Asparagus
- ❏ Beans: green, Italian, wax
- ❏ Bean sprouts
- ❏ Beets
- ❏ Broccoli
- ❏ Broccoli rabe
- ❏ Brussels sprouts
- ❏ Cabbage: bok choy, Chinese, green
- ❏ Carrots
- ❏ Cauliflower
- ❏ Celery
- ❏ Collard greens
- ❏ Cucumbers
- ❏ Eggplant
- ❏ Green onions (or scallions)
- ❏ Leeks
- ❏ Lettuce and salad greens
- ❏ Mung beans
- ❏ Mushrooms
- ❏ Mustard greens
- ❏ Okra
- ❏ Onions
- ❏ Peppers
- ❏ Radishes
- ❏ Sauerkraut
- ❏ Sea vegetables
- ❏ Spinach
- ❏ Swiss chard
- ❏ Turnips
- ❏ Turnip greens
- ❏ Water chestnuts
- ❏ Zucchini

Starchy Vegetables

❑ Corn

❑ Legumes (black beans, kidney beans, chickpeas, lentils, red beans)

❑ Parsnips

❑ Peas

❑ Plantains

❑ Potatoes

❑ Pumpkin

❑ Squash

❑ Yams

❑ Yucca

Lower-Carb Fruits

❑ Berries (raspberries, blackberries, strawberries, blueberries, cranberries)

❑ Cantaloupe

❑ Cherries

❑ Clementines

❑ Figs

❑ Grapefruit

❑ Guava

❑ Kiwi

❑ Lemon

❑ Lime

❑ Nectarine

❑ Papaya

❑ Peaches

❑ Plums

❑ Rhubarb

❑ Tangerine

❑ Tomatoes

Higher-Carb Fruits

❑ Apple

❑ Apricot

❑ Banana

❑ Dried fruits

❑ Grapes

❑ Mango

❑ Oranges

❑ Pear

❏ Pineapple

❏ Pomegranate

❏ Watermelon

Seafood

❏ Anchovies

❏ Bass

❏ Cod

❏ Grouper

❏ Halibut

❏ Herring

❏ Mackerel

❏ Mahi mahi

❏ Red snapper

❏ Salmon

❏ Sardines

❏ Shrimp

❏ Tuna

Meat

❏ Bacon (turkey or pork)

❏ Beef

❏ Bison

❏ Burgers: beef, chicken, turkey

❏ Chicken

❏ Duck

❏ Eggs

❏ Ground meat: chicken, turkey, beef

❏ Lamb

❏ Pork

❏ Sausages

❏ Sliced deli meat (be sure to heat it to avoid potential listeria contamination)

❏ Turkey

❏ Venison

Non-Animal Protein

- ❑ Tempeh (healthier alternative to tofu)
- ❑ Whey

Dairy/Nondairy

- ❑ Butter
- ❑ Cream (regular or heavy whipping)
- ❑ Cheese (feta, goat, cottage, Pecorino Romano, ricotta, cheddar, provolone, mozzarella)
- ❑ Ghee
- ❑ Mayonnaise
- ❑ Nondairy milk, unsweetened (almond, coconut, cashew)
- ❑ Nondairy yogurt (almond or coconut)
- ❑ Yogurt, plain Greek

Nuts and Seeds

- ❑ Almonds
- ❑ Brazil nuts
- ❑ Chia seeds
- ❑ Flax seeds
- ❑ Hazelnuts
- ❑ Hemp seeds
- ❑ Macadamia
- ❑ Nut butters: peanut, almond, cashew
- ❑ Pecans
- ❑ Pine nuts
- ❑ Pistachios
- ❑ Pumpkin seeds
- ❑ Quinoa
- ❑ Sunflower seeds
- ❑ Sunflower seed butter
- ❑ Sesame seeds
- ❑ Walnuts

Oil

❑ Almond

❑ Avocado

❑ Coconut

❑ Grapeseed

❑ Olive

❑ Sesame

❑ Walnut

Grains

❑ Amaranth

❑ Barley

❑ Bulgur

❑ Ezekiel bread

❑ Faro

❑ Millet

❑ Muesli

❑ Oats

❑ Pastas: black bean, red lentil, brown rice, chickpea, Einkorn

❑ Rice (brown, wild)

❑ Spelt

❑ Teff

❑ Tortillas (sprouted grain)

Spices and Herbs

❑ Basil

❑ Black pepper

❑ Cayenne pepper

❑ Chili pepper

❑ Cilantro

❑ Cinnamon

❑ Cloves

❑ Coriander seeds

❑ Cumin

❑ Dill

❑ Fennel

❑ Garlic

❑ Ginger

❑ Mint

❑ Mustard seeds

❑ Nutmeg

❑ Oregano

❑ Paprika

❑ Parsley

❑ Peppermint

❑ Pink Himalayan salt

❑ Rosemary

❑ Sage

❑ Tarragon

❑ Thyme

❑ Turmeric

Condiments

❑ Apple cider vinegar

❑ Balsamic vinegar

❑ Coconut amino acids

❑ Extracts (vanilla/almond)

❑ Guacamole

❑ Honey

❑ Hummus

❑ Mustard

❑ Lakanto maple syrup

❑ Salsa

❑ Stevia and other alternative sweeteners

❑ Tamari

Recommended Brands

- Bacon (turkey or pork): Applegate

- Butter: Kerrygold

- Barbecue sauce: Annie's

- Canned salmon, tuna, or chicken: Wild Planet

- Cheese slices: Applegate

- Chocolate chips: Lily's

- Crackers: Mary's Gone, GG Scandinavian Fiber Crispbread Crackers

- Flour (coconut): Bob's Red Mill

- Heavy whipping cream: Horizon Organic

  - Pancake mix: Bob's Red Mill

  - Pasta: Banza Chickpea Pasta

  - Tortillas: Food for Life Ezekiel 4:9 Organic Sprouted Grain Tortillas or Corn Tortillas (found in freezer aisle; store in fridge)

  - Mayonnaise: Sir Kensington or Primal Foods

  - Stevia

  - Swerve Confectioners (a good sugar replacement that doesn't have the bitter aftertaste of Stevia that some people dislike. Although the Nutrition Facts label reads 3 grams of carbohydrates, erythritol does not impact blood sugar levels.)

  - Lakanto maple syrup sweetened by monk fruit

  - Truvia

References

American Diabetes Association. "What Is Gestational Diabetes?" November 21, 2016. http://www.diabetes.org/diabetes-basics/gestational/what-is-gestational-diabetes.html

American Pregnancy Association. "Vitamin D and Pregnancy." April 3, 2017. http://americanpregnancy.org/pregnancy-health/vitamin-d-and-pregnancy.

Center for Food Safety and Applied Nutrition. "Labeling & Nutrition—Changes to the Nutrition Facts Label." United States Food and Drug Administration. June 28, 2018. https://www.fda.gov/Food/GuidanceRegulation/GuidanceDocumentsRegulatoryInformation/LabelingNutrition/ucm385663.htm#highlights.

Kampmann, Ulla, Lene Madsen, Gitte Skajaa, et al. "Gestational Diabetes: A Clinical Update." *World Journal of Diabetes* 6, no. 8 (2015): 1065–1072. doi: 10.4239/wjd.v6.i8.1065.

Osorio-Yáñez, Citlalli, Chunfang Qiu, Bizu Gelaye, et al. "Risk of Gestational Diabetes Mellitus in Relation to Maternal Dietary Calcium Intake." *Public Health Nutrition* 20, no. 6 (2017): 1082–1089. doi: 10.1017/S1368980016002974.

Padayachee, Cliantha and Jeff S. Coombes. "Exercise Guidelines for Gestational Diabetes Mellitus." *World Journal of Diabetes* 6, no. 8 (2015): 1033–1044. doi: 10.4239/wjd.v6.i8.1033.

Pan, Mei-Lien, Li-Ru Chen, Hsiao-Mei Tsao, et al. "Relationship between Polycystic Ovarian Syndrome and Subsequent Gestational Diabetes Mellitus: A Nationwide Population-Based Study." *PLoS ONE* 10, no. 10 (2015): e0140544. doi: 10.1371/journal.pone.0140544.

Racusin, Diana, Nelli Crawford, Sara Andrabi, et al. "Twizzlers as a Cost-Effective and Equivalent Alternative to the Glucola Beverage in Diabetes Screening." *Diabetes Care* 36, no. 10 (2013): e169–e170. doi: 10.2337/dc13-1130.

Saudan, Patrick, Mark Brown, Megan Buddle, et al. "Does Gestational Hypertension Become Pre-eclampsia?" *British Journal of Obstetrics and Gynaecology,* 105, no. 11 (1998): 1177–1184. doi: 10.1111/j.1471-0528.1998.tb09971.x.

Schaub, Eve. "The Sugar Alphabet: 54 Different Names for Sugar." EveSchaub.com. May 12, 2014. https://eveschaub.com/2014/05/12/the-sugar-alphabet-54-different-names-for-sugar

Conversion Charts

Volume Conversions

U.S.	U.S. Equivalent	Metric
1 tablespoon (3 teaspoons)	½ fluid oz	15 ml
¼ cup	2 fluid oz	60 ml
⅓ cup	3 fluid oz	90 ml
½ cup	4 fluid 0z	120 ml
⅔ cup	5 fluid oz	150 ml
¾ cup	6 fluid oz	180 ml
1 cup	8 fluid oz	240 ml
2 cups	16 fluid oz	480 ml

Weight Conversions

U.S.	Metric
½ ounce	15 grams
1 ounce	30 grams
2 ounces	60 grams
¼ pound	115 grams
⅓ pound	150 grams
½ pound	225 grams
¾ pound	350 grams
1 pound	450 grams

Temperature Conversions

Fahrenheit (°F)	Celsius (°C)
70°F	20°C
100°F	40°C
120°F	50°C
130°F	55°C
140°F	60°C
150°F	65°C
160°F	70°C
170°F	75°C
180°F	80°C
190°F	90°C
200°F	95°C
220°F	105°C
240°F	115°C
260°F	125°C
280°F	140°C
300°F	150°C
325°F	165°C
350°F	175°C
375°F	190°C
400°F	200°C
425°F	220°C
450°F	230°C

Recipe Index

About the Author

Sara Rivera is a registered dietitian based in New Jersey. She has dedicated her life to spreading awareness of real food nutrition to help people find freedom from chronic health conditions and harmful dieting. Sara is the founder of her private practice, Mindful Meals Nutrition Services, LLC, where patients with a variety of nutrition-related diseases are provided with medical nutrition therapy, education, and meal preparation services. Sara is also the coauthor of *DASH Diet for Renal Health*.

To learn more, please visit: www.dietitiansara.com.